Animal Cell Culture and Technology

Second Edition

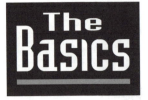

Series Advisors:

Rob Beynon UMIST, Manchester, UK
Chris Howe Department of Biochemistry, University of Cambridge, Cambridge, UK

Monoclonal Antibodies
PCR
Analyzing Chromosomes
Separating Cells
Biological Centrifugation
Plant Cell Culture
Animal Cell Culture and Technology

Forthcoming titles

Analyzing Gene Expression
Gene Mapping
Reconstructing Evolutionary Trees

Animal Cell Culture and Technology

Second Edition

Michael Butler

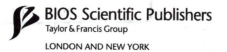

BIOS Scientific Publishers

Taylor & Francis Group

LONDON AND NEW YORK

© Garland Science/BIOS Scientific Publishers, 2004

First published 2004

A CIP catalogue record for this book is available from the British Library.

ISBN 1 859960499

Garland Science/BIOS Scientific Publishers
4 Park Square, Milton Park, Abingdon, Oxon, OX14 4RN, UK and
29 West 35th Street, New York, NY 10001–2299, USA
World Wide Web home page: www.bios.co.uk

Garland Science/BIOS Scientific Publishers is a member of the Taylor & Francis Group.

Distributed in the USA by
Fulfilment Center
Taylor & Francis
10650 Toebben Drive
Independence, KY 41051, USA
Toll Free Tel.: +1 800 634 7064; E-mail: taylorandfrancis@thomsonlearning.com

Distributed in Canada by
Taylor & Francis
74 Rolark Drive
Scarborough, Ontario M1R 4G2, Canada
Toll Free Tel.: +1 877 226 2237; E-mail: tal_fran@istar.ca

Distributed in the rest of the world by
Thomson Publishing Services
Cheriton House
North Way
Andover, Hampshire SP10 5BE, UK
Tel.: +44 (0)1264 332424; E-mail: salesorder.tandf@thomsonpublishingservices.co.uk

Production Editor: Georgia Bushell
Typeset by J&L Composition, Filey, North Yorkshire UK
Printed and bound by TJ International, Padstow, Cornwall UK

The Basics

Contents

Chapter 4 Growth and maintenance of cells in culture   47

Chapter 5 Cell line and culture monitoring   67

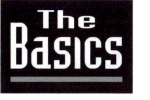

used in commercial bioprocesses, but in other cases they are included to show what alternatives could be considered.

Viral vaccines represented the major group of commercial products from mammalian cell cultures for years. These are generally produced from well-defined anchorage-dependent cells grown in microcarriers. However, there is now a growing list of other important commercial products such as monoclonal antibodies and recombinant proteins that have been licensed for human therapeutic use. Monoclonal antibodies can now be 'humanized' by appropriate molecular recombination of mouse antibodies and human immunoglobulin regions. This has created a huge potential for the use of antibodies in the treatment of human disease. These developments account for the growing expansion of the biotechnology industry and the need for increased capacity for large-scale cell culture bioprocesses. The demand for biomanufacturing is predicted to increase even further as generic copies of the originally patented biological molecules are allowed.

The commercial developments of animal cell technology can be followed through the archives of two major conference groups – the European Society of Animal Cell Technology (ESACT) and the Cell Culture Engineering (CCE) meetings. These organizations host meetings on alternate years and each has become a showcase for the biotechnology industry and the cell culture technology that underpins it. The increasing demand for attendance at these meetings is evidence of the growing expansion of the technology. The subject area has also become popular at universities as the demand for expertise in the technology is high and can be translated to good work prospects for students. The course in Industrial Microbiology at the University of Manitoba is one such course that includes a high content of the material outlined in this book

It is hoped that this book may act as an easily readable introduction to animal cell culture and technology to undergraduates, graduates, technicians or experienced industrial researchers who are about to start projects or courses involving the use of cell culture. The explanations are kept basic, in keeping with the rest of the series, so that the minimal amount of background knowledge is assumed. In this way, it is hoped that even those students with little background in the biological sciences may find this information useful.

Michael Butler
University of Manitoba
September 2003

Chapter 1

The Basics

Introduction: The use of animal cell culture

1. Tissue culture, organ culture and cell culture

Cells, removed from animal tissue or whole animals, will continue to grow if supplied with nutrients and growth factors. This process is called cell culture. It occurs *in vitro* ('in glass') as opposed to *in vivo* ('in life'). The culture process allows single cells to act as independent units much like any microorganism such as bacteria or fungi. The cells are capable of division by mitosis and the cell population can continue growth until limited by some parameter such as nutrient depletion.

Animal cells selected for culture are maintained as independent units. Cultures normally contain cells of one type (e.g. fibroblasts). The cells in the culture may be genetically identical (homogeneous population) or may show some genetic variation (heterogeneous population). A homogeneous population of cells derived from a single parental cell is called a clone. Therefore all cells within a clonal population are genetically identical. Cell culture is a widely used technique and is the main subject of this book.

Cell culture is quite different from organ culture. Organ culture means the maintenance of whole organs or fragments of tissue with the retention of a balanced relationship between the associated cell types as exists *in vivo*. This idea of the maintenance of tissue was important in the early development of culture techniques. However, it was soon realized that this was extremely difficult over long periods because of the differing growth potential of individual cell types within a tissue.

Nowadays the culture of individual cells is the preferred technique because conditions can be controlled to allow some degree of consistency and reproducibility in cell growth. Although 'cell culture' is the most appropriate and logical term for this, it is still widely referred to as 'tissue culture' – a term that can be misleading, as it is also used to refer to organ culture.

2. Why grow animal cells in culture?

There are a number of applications for animal cell cultures:

- to investigate the normal physiology or biochemistry of cells. For example, metabolic pathways can be investigated by applying radioactively labeled substrates and subsequently looking at products;
- to test the effects of compounds on specific cell types. Such compounds may be metabolites, hormones or growth factors. Similarly, potentially toxic or mutagenic compounds may be evaluated in cell culture;
- to produce artificial tissue by combining specific cell types in sequence. This has considerable potential for production of artificial skin for use in treatment of burns.

■   to synthesize valuable products (biologicals) from large-scale cell cultures. The biologicals encompass a broad range of cell products and include specific proteins or viruses that require animal cells for propagation. The number of such commercially valuable biologicals has increased rapidly over the last decade and has led to the present widespread interest in animal cell technology. Proteins that are present in minute quantities *in vivo* can be synthesized in gram (or kilogram) quantities by growing genetically engineered cells *in vitro*.

3.   The advantages and disadvantages of using cell culture

In all the situations listed above we could use animal tissue (e.g. liver) or whole animals (e.g. mice). Biochemists have traditionally used homogenized liver as a source of cells for enzyme or metabolic studies. So, why use animal cell culture which may require far more time in preparation and may require specialized equipment?

The major advantage to using cell culture is the consistency and reproducibility of results that can be obtained by using a batch of cells of a single type and preferably a homogeneous population (clonal). For example, we may be doing a biochemical analysis where it is important to relate a particular metabolic pathway to a certain cell type. This would be possible in a culture containing a homogeneous cell population which can be monitored for biochemical and genetic characteristics, but very difficult in a tissue homogenate which would contain a heterogeneous mix of cells at different stages of growth and viability.

Toxicological testing procedures have been well established in laboratory animals. However, the use of cell culture techniques may allow a greater understanding of the effects of a particular compound on a specific cell type such as liver cells (hepatocytes). Furthermore, routine toxicity tests are far less expensive in cell culture than in whole animals.

In the production of biological products on a large scale, the avoidance of contaminants such as unwanted viruses or proteins is important. This can be more easily performed in a well-characterized cell culture than when dealing with pooled animal tissue.

The major disadvantage to the use of cell culture is that after a period of continuous growth, cell characteristics can change and may be quite different from those originally found in the donor animal. Cells can adapt to different nutrients. This adaptation involves changes in intracellular enzyme activities. Furthermore, culturing favors the survival of fast-growing cells which are selectively retained in a mixed cell population.

The changes in the growth and biochemical characteristics of a cell population may be a particular problem when using cultures to develop an understanding of the behavior of cells *in vivo*. After a period of culture, the cells may be significantly different from those that are highly differentiated *in vivo* where growth has ceased. Intracellular enzyme activities change dramatically in response to nutrient depletion and by-product accumulation in a culture.

Some of the characteristics of cells in culture are discussed further in Chapter 2.

4. The early history of cell culture

The techniques necessary to allow animal cells to grow in culture were gradually developed over the course of the last century (see *Table 1.1*). The original impetus for the development of cell culture was to study, under a microscope, normal physiological events such as nerve development.

One of the earliest experiments showing cell culture *in vitro* was conducted by Ross Harrison in 1907 who developed the 'hanging drop' technique which is illustrated in *Figure 1.1*. In the depression of a microscope slide he entrapped small pieces of frog embryo tissue in clotted lymph fluid (Harrison, 1907). By this method he was able to observe the elongation of nerve fibers over several weeks.

From his experiments he demonstrated some of the characteristics and requirements for the maintenance of cells.

Table 1.1. Milestones in the development of animal cell technology

Year	Milestone
1880	
	Roux maintained embryonic chick cells in saline solution
1890	
1900	
	Harrison grew frog nerve cells by the 'hanging drop' technique
1910	
	Carrel used aseptic techniques for long-term cell cultures
	Rous and Jones used trypsin for subculture of adherent cells
1920	
	The 'Carrel' flask was designed for cell culture
1930	
1940	
	Antibiotics were added to culture medium
	Earle isolated mouse L fibroblasts
	Enders grew polio virus on cultured human cells
1950	
	Gey cultured HeLa cells
	Eagle developed a chemically defined culture medium
1960	
	Hayflick and Moorhead showed that human cells have a finite lifespan
	Ham grew cells in a serum-free medium
	Harris and Watkins fused human and mice cells
1970	
	Kohler and Milstein produced an antibody-secreting hybridoma
	Sato developed serum-free media from hormones and growth factors
1980	
	Human insulin was produced from bacteria
	Monoclonal antibody (OKT3) used for human therapy
	Recombinant tPA licensed for human therapy
1990	
	Humanized chimeric antibodies used for human therapy
	Stem cells isolated

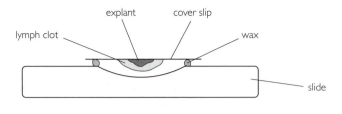

Figure 1.1

Hanging drop technique of cell culture.

- The cells require an anchor for support which in this case was provided by the coverslip and the fibrous matrix of the lymph clot. Cells that are bound to a tissue matrix *in vivo* are normally anchorage-dependent when grown in culture. Several proteins are responsible for glueing the cells to a solid surface. The best characterized is fibronectin.
- The cells require nutrients which are provided by the biological fluid contained in the clot.
- The growth rate is relatively slow (compared to bacteria) and this makes the culture vulnerable to contamination. A small number of bacteria would soon outgrow a larger population of animal cells. The doubling time for animal cells is normally between 18 and 24 hours but bacterial cells can double in 30 minutes.

Some of these early culture experiments were continued by Alexis Carrel who was trained as a surgeon (Carrel, 1912). He showed that the application of strict aseptic control enabled the prolonged subculture of the cells. He used chick embryo extracts mixed with blood plasma to support cell growth. In 1923 Carrel designed a flask suitable for routine cell culture work (*Figure 1.2*). This facilitated subculture under aseptic conditions and was the fore-runner of the modern cell culture flask. Sterile manipulation is facilitated by the narrow-angled glass neck of the Carrel flask which can be flamed by a Bunsen burner prior to inoculation or sampling.

However, Carrel's application of surgical procedures for aseptic manipu-lation of cell cultures was elaborate and difficult to repeat by others. Consequently cell culture was not adopted as a routine laboratory technique until much later (reviewed by Witkowski, 1979). Of course, today cell culture is widely used and can be performed in most moderately equipped laboratories.

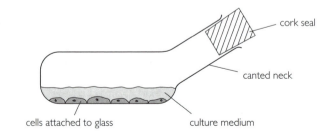

Figure 1.2

The Carrel flask.

Carrel is particularly well known for his 34-year culture experiment. In 1912 he isolated a population of chick embryo fibroblasts and these cells were grown in culture until 1946. From this, Carrel concluded that the cells were immortal. However, this claim was later refuted by the work of Hayflick and Moorhead who showed the finite lifespan of isolated animal cells (see below). It is now thought that Carrel's technique of using plasma and homogenized tissue as growth medium most likely allowed continuous re-inoculation of cells into his culture.

5.   How long will primary cultures survive?

In 1961, Hayflick and Moorhead studied the growth potential of human embryonic cells. They showed that these cells could be grown continuously through repeated subculture for about 50 generations (Hayflick and Moorhead, 1961). After this time, the cells enter a senescent phase and are incapable of further growth. *Figure 1.3* illustrates the pattern of growth during the lifespan of these cells.

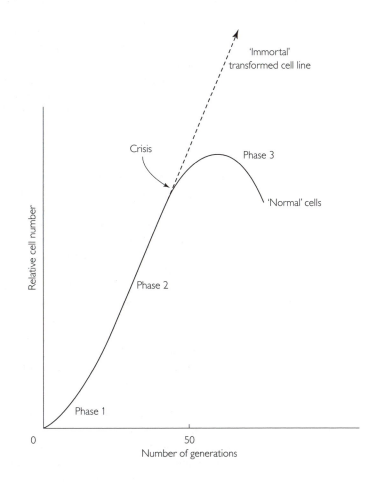

Figure 1.3

Normal and transformed growth of human embryonic cells over an extended number of passages.

A finite growth capacity is a characteristic of all cells derived from normal animal tissue. The cells appear to pass through a series of age-related changes until the final stage when the cells are incapable of dividing further. The finite number of generations of growth is a characteristic of the cell type, age and species of origin and is referred to as the 'Hayflick limit'.

The capacity for growth is related to the origin of the cells – those derived from embryonic tissue have a greater growth capacity than those derived from adult tissue. Each cell appears to have an inherent 'biological clock' defined by the number of divisions from the original stem cell. Even if cells are stored by cryopreservation the total capacity for cell division is not altered.

6.   The biological clock

The molecular mechanism that limits the growth capacity of normal cells was a mystery for a number of years until some key observations were made regarding chromosomal length. In 1986 Howard Cooke made the observation that the caps at the end of chromosomes of human germline cells were longer than somatic cells (Cooke and Smith, 1986). These caps known as telomeres are repeats of the nucleotide sequence TTAGGG/CCCTAA and are shortened at each generation of growth of somatic cells. This is not surprising given the semiconservative mechanism of DNA replication which operates in one direction (5′ to 3′ end). This generates a fork of replication that cannot work at the end of double-stranded DNA. Therefore, at each mitotic division there is a small segment of DNA that is not replicated, thus shortening the telomeric cap.

However, in germ cells the telomere is maintained at 15 kilobases apparently by a ribonucleoprotein enzyme, telomerase. The telomerase is expressed in germ cells and has moderate activity in stem cells but is absent in somatic cells. The finite lifespan of normal somatic cells is regulated by 10 or more 'senescence' genes that suppress the expression of the telomerase gene. This causes the human telomeres to gradually shorten at a rate of around 100 basepairs per cell division. From the telomere hypothesis, cells become senescent and stop dividing when progressive telomeric shortening produces a threshold telomere length. If oncogenes are activated then cells escape the negative control of the cell cycle and re-express telomerase.

The critical experiment to validate this hypothesis came with a publication in 1998. Bodnar *et al.* (1998) described the introduction of human telomerase reverse transcriptase (hTRT) into normal human cells (retinal pigment epithelial cells and foreskin fibroblasts). This converted the normal hTRT$^-$ state to hTRT$^+$ with the capability for expression of the telomerase enzyme. This process succeeded in increasing the lifespan of the cells significantly. The mean population doubling capacity of both cell types increased by at least 20 generations. *Figure 1.4* shows that for clones of the epithelial cells the mean population doubling of 54 generations increased to a value of 73 generations by the introduction of the telomerase enzyme. Similarly, for the fibroblasts, there was an increase of the mean population doubling of 64 to 100. This experiment established a causal relationship between telomere shortening and *in vitro* cell senescence which is dependent upon a mitotic clock.

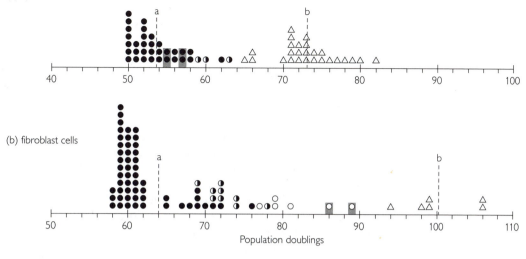

Figure 1.4

The effect of telomerase activity on the growth span of cells. The initial mean doubling time (a) of the cell clones was extended (b) by the introduction of the telomerase gene. Modified from Bodnar et al., 1998.

7. The first products of animal cell technology

The impetus for the application of cell culture to large-scale production came with the need for viral vaccines. Major epidemics of polio in the 1940s and 1950s prompted a lot of effort to develop an effective vaccine. In 1949, Enders showed that the poliomyelitis virus could be grown in cultures of human embryonic cells (Enders *et al.*, 1949). The polio vaccine, which could be produced from the de-activated virus, became one of the first commercial products of cultured animal cells. Initially the virus was propagated on primary cells, which are defined as those taken directly from an animal into culture. Later primary monkey kidney cells were replaced by human diploid lung fibroblast cells with defined characteristics (e.g. WI-38, MRC-5). These were widely accepted because of their apparent 'normality'. Since the 1950s a range of human and veterinary vaccines have been produced routinely from large-scale mammalian cell cultures.

During the 1950s, several cell types with good growth characteristics were isolated and characterized. These included the chemically transformed mouse L cells and the human carcinoma cell line, HeLa, which derives from the name of the donor – Henrietta Lach, although some texts designate the name as Helen Lane. Earle and Eagle focused their attention on the development of chemically defined nutrient formulations for the growth of these cells and to replace the undefined biological extracts previously used (Eagle, 1955). The chemically defined media, Eagle's Minimum Essential Medium (EMEM) developed in the 1950s was the first widely used culture medium. EMEM had several advantages over previously used media:

■ consistency between culture batches;
■ ease of sterilization;
■ reduced chance of contamination.

Basic research in the 1960s using cell culture techniques included the classical work of Hayflick and Moorhead which is described in Section 5 of this chapter. This established that there is a finite lifespan intrinsic to the genetic make-up of all normal animal cells.

Recombinant DNA technology was developed in the 1970s. This allowed DNA to be isolated and inserted in any cell. Initially this was used for the expression of mammalian genes in bacteria (particularly *E. coli*). It was considered at the time that such genetically engineered bacteria could be developed for the production of any desired mammalian protein. However, it soon became apparent that large complex proteins (particularly those with carbohydrate groups attached) could only be synthesized with all their post-translational modifications in eukaryotic cells. Bacteria do not have the appropriate metabolism to complete these modifications which are necessary for full activity of many mammalian proteins. Therefore, genetically engineered animal cells were developed for the large-scale commercial synthesis of such important complex macromolecules as plasminogen activator, factor VIII and erythropoietin. These compounds have been licensed for human therapeutic use.

Fusion techniques were pioneered in the 1960s by Harris and Watkins who allowed cells of different origin to be fused to produce hybrids. The initial value of this work was to be able to assign specific genes to specific chromosomes. However, a novel application of this fusion technique was described by Kohler and Milstein in 1975 who produced hybridoma cells capable of the continuous production of a single type of antibody (Kohler and Milstein, 1975). These monoclonal antibodies have been particularly valued as diagnostic and therapeutic agents because of their ability to selectively bind specific compounds. They are now produced commercially in kilogram quantities from the large-scale culture of hybridomas.

The three major categories of valuable products from animal cells that we can identify over the last 40 years are:

- viral vaccines;
- monoclonal antibodies;
- recombinant glycoproteins.

The range of these biologicals has increased rapidly over the last few years. This is particularly so for the glycoproteins that are of use as pharmaceutical, medical or veterinary products. They are generally synthesized as secreted products from selected or genetically engineered mammalian cell lines. They are needed in large quantities and this requires a careful study of the control of the production processes. Such a study should start with an examination of the principles of biochemistry, cell biology and biochemical engineering that underlie such production processes.

References

Bodnar, A.G., Ouellette, M., Frolkis, M., Holt, S.E., Chiu, C.-P., Morin, G.B., Harley, C.B., Shay, J.W., Lichtsteiner, S. and Wright, W.E. (1998) Extension of life-span by introduction of telomerase into normal human cells. *Science* 279: 349–352.

Carrel, A. (1912) On the permanent life of tissues outside the organism. *J. Exp. Med.* 15: 516–528.

Cooke, H.J. and Smith, B.A. (1986) Variability at the telomeres of the human X/Y pseudoautosomal region. *Cold Spring Harbor Symp. Quant. Biol.* **51 Pt1:** 213–219.

Eagle, H. (1955) Nutrition needs of mammalian cells in tissue culture. *Science* **122:** 501–504.

Enders, J.F., Weller, T.H. and Robbins, F.C. (1949) Cultivation of the Lansing strain of poliomyelitis virus in cultures of various human embryonic tissues. *Science* **109:** 85–87.

Harrison, R.G. (1907) Observations on the living developing nerve fibre. *Proc. Soc. Exp. Biol. Med.* **4:** 140–143.

Hayflick, L. and Moorhead, P.S. (1961) The serial cultivation of human diploid cell strains. *Exp. Cell Res.* **25:** 585–621.

Kohler, G. and Milstein, C. (1975) Continuous culture of fused cells secreting antibody of predefined specificity. *Nature* (London) **256:** 495–497.

Witkowski, J.A. (1979) Alexis Carrel and the mysticism of tissue culture. *Med. Hist.* **23:** 270–296.

Further reading

The first few chapters of the following texts provide a good historical and theoretical background to the subject.

Paul, J. (1975) *Cell and Tissue Culture.* Churchill Livingstone, Edinburgh.

Sharp, J.A. (1977) *An Introduction to Animal Tissue Culture.* E. Arnold, London.

Spier, R.E. and Griffiths, J.B. (eds) (1985) *Animal Cell Technology,* Vol. 1. Academic Press, London.

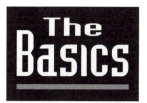

Chapter 2

Characteristics of cells in culture

1. Where to obtain cells?

A major choice has to be made when establishing a cell culture as to whether cells are obtained directly from animal tissue or from a culture collection. The choice will depend upon what the objective of the project is and the nature of the experiments planned. Isolation directly from tissue offers a means of culturing cells close to their state *in vivo*. However, the isolation process is far more demanding and troublesome compared to establishing a culture from a cell sample that could be obtained from a culture collection. Most culture laboratories prefer to use cell lines from collections because they are well characterized in terms of growth, origin and genetic traits.

2. Cells from tissue: a primary culture

A primary culture is established when the cells taken directly from animal tissue are added to growth medium. Primary cultures are often established from embryonic tissue because the cells are more easily dispersed and have a superior growth potential. The structure of a tissue is highly ordered and comprises a range of cell types as shown for the cross-section of the epidermis shown in *Figure 2.1*. The objective of establishing a primary culture is to select a single cell type from this ordered structure.

The original methods developed for tissue culture by Harrison and Carrel involved the maintenance of tissue fragments (or explant) on a solid surface and supplied with suitable nutrients. However, such cultures are of greater use if the individual cells are separated out before culture. This is done by fragmenting tissue with forceps and scissors followed by treatment with a proteolytic enzyme such as trypsin or collagenase. The proteolytic action of the enzymes disaggregates the tissue into individual cells after which the cells are isolated by low-speed centrifugation. The time that the cells are in contact with the degradative enzymes should be minimized otherwise membrane damage may occur. Cells can be bathed in trypsin for 10–20 minutes. Longer exposure times are undesirable because breakdown of the protein components of cell membranes could occur. Collagenase degrades collagen and is less harmful to cell membranes.

This technique works well for most tissues although some modifications to the general procedure may be necessary to ensure the maximum yield of a particular cell type. One of the major difficulties and reasons for failure at this stage is that the cell population becomes contaminated with bacteria or fungi (see Chapter 4). To avoid this problem it is important to maintain aseptic techniques throughout the process of establishing the primary culture. All the dissection instruments should be sterile and all working

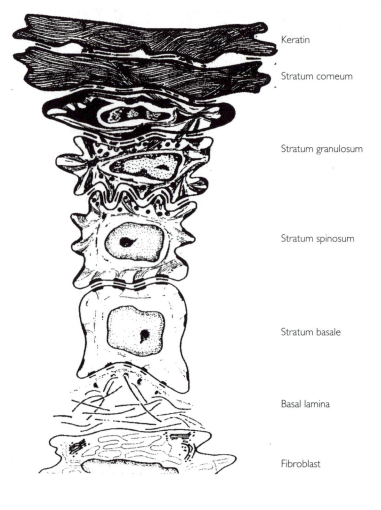

Keratin

Stratum corneum

Stratum granulosum

Stratum spinosum

Stratum basale

Basal lamina

Fibroblast

Figure 2.1

Ordered cell layers in the epidermis. Modified from Fusening, 1986.

surfaces should be swabbed with 70% alcohol. A typical protocol for obtaining a primary culture of chick embryo fibroblasts is described at the end of the chapter (*Protocol 2.1*).

When the cells in a primary culture stop growing a new culture may be established by inoculating some of the cells into fresh medium. This is called subculturing or passaging (see Chapter 4). A secondary culture is established after the first passage of the primary culture. The term 'cell line' is applied to the cell population that can continue growing through many subcultures. However it should be noted that the greatest chance of genetic alteration occurs in the first few passages following the primary culture as cells adapt to a new chemical environment. The chick embryo fibroblasts may grow for around 30 passages before becoming senescent. The passage number of a culture is often recorded as the number of subcultures from the primary source.

3. Cell types

Animal cells are usually defined by the tissue from which they have derived and have characteristic shapes that can be observed and recognized easily through a light microscope. *Figure 2.2* illustrates the morphology of the cells commonly grown in culture. These are derived from five main types of animal tissue.

- Epithelial tissue consists of a layer of cells which cover organs and line cavities; examples include skin and the lining of the alimentary canal. The epithelial cells grow well in culture as a single cell monolayer and have a characteristic cobble-stone appearance.

- Connective tissue forms a major structural component of animals, consisting of a fibrous matrix and including bone cartilage. The tissue contains fibroblasts which are amongst the most widely used cells in laboratory cultures. Fibroblasts are bound to the fibrous protein collagen in the connective tissue. The cells are spherical when first dissociated by trypsin from the tissue but elongate to a characteristic spindle-shape on attachment to a solid surface. Fibroblasts have excellent growth characteristics and have been the 'favorite' cells for establishing cultures. Fibroblast and epithelial cells adapt relatively easily to culture and have growth rates with a doubling time of 18–24 hours. *Figure 2.3* shows a high magnification electron micrograph of fibroblasts associated with a collagen matrix.

- Muscle tissue consists of a series of tubules formed from precursor cells which fuse to form a multinucleate complex and which also contain the structural proteins (actin and myosin). The precursor cells are myoblasts which are capable of differentiation to form myotubes – a

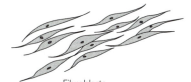
Fibroblasts

Epithelial cells

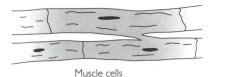
Muscle cells

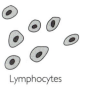
Lymphocytes

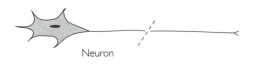
Neuron

0   20 µm

Figure 2.2

Cell types commonly used in culture.

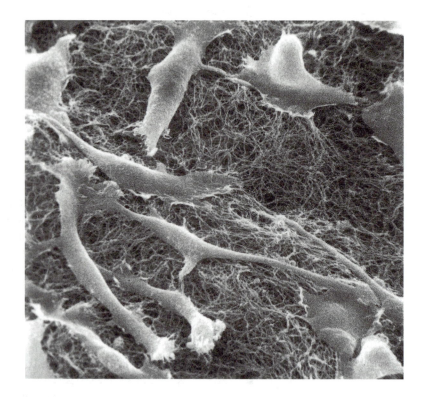

Figure 2.3

Scanning electron micrograph of bovine fibroblast cells on a collagen matrix (×1800).

process that can be observed in culture. *Figure 2.2* shows the myoblast alignment that occurs during the process.

■ Nervous tissue consists of characteristically shaped neurons which are responsible for the transmission of electrical impulses and supporting cells, such as glial cells. Neurons are highly differentiated and have not been observed to divide in culture. However, the addition of nerve growth factor to cultures of neurons may cause the formation of cytoplasmic outgrowths called neurites. Some of the characteristics of nerve cells can be observed with neuroblastomas which are tumor cells that undergo cell growth in culture.

■ Blood and lymph contain a range of cells in suspension. Some of these will continue growth in a culture suspension. These include the lymphoblasts which are white blood cells and are used extensively in culture because of their ability to secrete immunoregulating compounds.

4.   How to select a particular cell type

The primary culture will almost certainly contain a variety of different cell types with differing growth capacities. However, for most experimental work it is important to isolate a single cell type from the culture population. There are several ways this can be achieved.

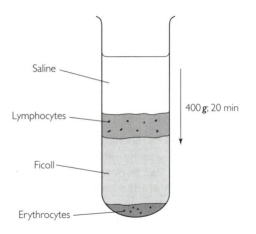

Figure 2.4

Separation of cells by density gradient centrifugation.

■ Allow the cells to grow. Fast-growing cell types may assume dominance in a population. For example, fibroblasts have relatively short population doubling times and may outgrow other cells after a few generations (called 'fibroblast overgrowth').

■ Control the composition of the growth medium. The addition of specific growth factors or known growth inhibitors may allow selective growth of certain cell types.

■ Separate cells by using gradient centrifugation (Sykes *et al.*, 1970). The cells sediment to an equilibrium position equivalent to their own density – a process called isopycnic sedimentation. The gradients can be formed by nontoxic, high-molecular-weight material such as colloidal silica as developed by Pharmacia in their formulations 'Ficoll' and 'Percoll'. This method is particularly effective for the isolation of certain cell types in sterile medium, for example lymphocytes from blood (*Protocol 2.2*). Cell separation by a simple gradient centrifugation process is shown in *Figure 2.4*.

5. What is a 'normal' cell?

In the 1960s, 'normal' mammalian cells were required as hosts for the production of human vaccines in order to ensure the safety of these products. In order to meet this requirement, a number of characteristics of 'normal' animal cells were defined by Hayflick and Moorhead following their work with human embryonic cells (see Chapter 1 Section 5):

■ a diploid chromosome number (e.g.: 46 chromosomes for human cells). This indicates that no gross chromosomal damage has occurred;

■ anchorage dependence. The cells require a solid substratum for attachment and growth. Growth continues until a confluent monolayer of cells is formed on the substratum;

■ a finite lifespan. This is a reflection of the intrinsic growth potential of the cells;

■ nonmalignant. The cells are not cancerous. This can be shown by the inability of the cells to form a tumor following injection into immuno-compromised mice.

6.   Anchorage-dependence

Anchorage-dependence is the requirement of cells for a solid substratum for attachment before growth can occur. At the laboratory scale this substratum can be provided by the solid surface of Petri dishes, T-flasks, or Roux bottles which are made of specially treated glass or plastic. The interaction between the cell membrane and the growth surface is critical and involves a combination of electrostatic attraction and van der Waal's forces. Cell adhesion occurs by divalent cations (usually Ca^{2+}) and basic proteins forming a layer between the solid substratum and the cell surface. In most cases the cell-surface interaction is provided by a range of nonspecific proteins which form a 2.5 nm-thick layer on the substratum prior to cell attachment.

Figure 2.5 outlines the process of cell attraction to the substratum and the involvement of various proteins in cell-surface bonding. Serum-derived glycoproteins (e.g. fibronectin) can provide a surface coating conducive to cell attachment. Conditioning factors are released by cells into the medium and help in forming a bond between cell surface glycoproteins and the substratum.

The density of the electrostatic charge on the solid substratum is also critical in maximizing cell attachment. A negative charge is provided on glass surface containers by alkali treatment. Tissue culture-grade plasticware consists of sulfonated polystyrene with a surface charge of 2–5 negatively charged groups per nm^2.

Culture systems are also available for the large-scale production of anchorage-dependent cells and are described in Chapter 9.

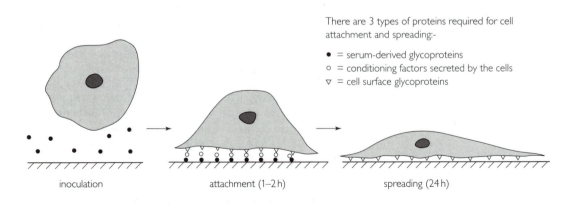

There are 3 types of proteins required for cell attachment and spreading:-

● = serum-derived glycoproteins
○ = conditioning factors secreted by the cells
▽ = cell surface glycoproteins

inoculation   attachment (1–2 h)   spreading (24 h)

Figure 2.5

The adhesion of anchorage-dependent cells to a solid substratum.

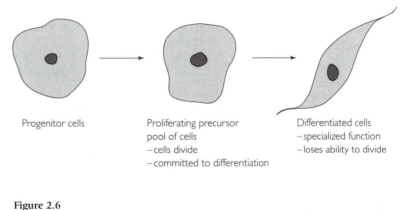

Progenitor cells

Proliferating precursor
pool of cells
–cells divide
–committed to differentiation

Differentiated cells
–specialized function
–loses ability to divide

Figure 2.6

Cell differentiation.

7.   The culture of differentiated cells

Differentiation is a process whereby cells slowly change their characteristics to become specialized cells with characteristic phenotypes. *Figure 2.6* outlines a typical sequence of changes that occurs during cell differentiation *in vivo*. This process occurs *in vivo* during embryo development or during wound healing and leads to the formation of cells with specialized function (differentiated) such as neurons or muscle cells. Differentiation is also associated with normal cell replacement, as is necessary in the bloodstream. The undifferentiated precursors of this process are called stem cells.

Most stem cells or embryonic cells grow well in culture. However, as cells become more specialized (differentiated) they tend to lose their growth capabilities and this is reflected by poor growth in culture. For most cell types proliferation is incompatible with the expression of differentiated properties.

However, when some cells derived from a tissue are placed in culture there can be an apparent loss in differentiated properties in the surviving cell population. Some explanation can be offered for this:

■   selective outgrowth of undifferentiated cell types. These include fibroblasts and epithelial cells that may be obtained from nongrowing animal tissue;

■   adaptive response of cells to the culture media.

Tumor cells are, in most cases, undifferentiated and have good growth characteristics. However, there are also some differentiated tumor cells which have proved extremely valuable. For example neuroblastomas are fast-growing tumor cells which have been used to study response effects with nerve growth factor.

Differentiated tumor cells retain the phenotypic characteristics of normal differentiated cells but are also able to grow in culture.

Although growth of most differentiated cells is poor, the following factors may allow some differentiated properties of normal cells to be maintained in culture.

- Hormones and growth factors. There are a number of media formulations containing selective components that can maintain the differentiated state of specific cell types, for example keratinocytes, hepatocytes and nerve cells.
- Chemical agents. Solvents such as dimethyl sulfoxide (DMSO) may allow the maintenance of a differentiated state by an effect on membrane fluidity.
- Cell interactions. Contact between cells may allow the formation of gap junctions and allow metabolites to synchronize the expression of differentiation within a cell population. This may also play a part in the arrest of growth when a cell population has covered an available growth surface (defined as 'confluence').
- Interaction with the growth surface. Collagen has been found to be essential for maintaining the polarity of hepatocytes in relation to the attachment surface. Cell polarity is governed by an asymmetrical distribution of ion currents (particularly Ca^{2+}). This allows one end of the cell to be functionally distinct from the other.

Some culture systems have been extremely valuable in investigating the metabolic changes that are associated with differentiation. However, growth in these cultures is either nonexistent or can be prolonged only for a short period (weeks).

8. Embryonic stem cells

These cells are capable of apparently unlimited growth but have the capacity, given the appropriate stimuli, to differentiate into any other cell type. Human embryonic stem cells were first isolated in 1998 by J. Thomson at the University of Wisconsin, who derived several cell lines and showed their capacity for growth for up to at least 300 population doublings (Thomson *et al.*, 1998). The cells were derived from the inner cell mass (~30 cells) of a human blastocyte formed from several days growth of an embryo following *in vitro* fertilization. These embryonic stem cells have been shown to have several important properties.

- Pluripotent. They have the capacity for differentiation into the cells of the three major tissue types (endoderm, mesoderm and ectoderm). This means that they have the potential to act as precursors for all cells of the body.
- They can be propagated indefinitely in a non-differentiated state.
- Directed differentiation. They can be induced to follow a specific pathway of differentiation, given the appropriate chemicals, growth factors or cell contact.
- They are associated with specific cell markers, e.g. Oct-4 transcription factor and stage-specific embryonic antigen (SSEA).
- They have a normal diploid karyotype.
- The cells have a high activity level of telomerase. This tends to correlate with immortality in human cell lines.
- If injected into immunocompromised mice they form a teratoma in which some of the major differentiated cell types can be distinguished.

8.1   Directed differentiation

If embryonic stem cells are allowed to clump then they form an embryoid body in which the cells begin to differentiate spontaneously. However, through directed differentiation the addition of specific growth factors may direct the cells down a specific pathway of change (Wichterle *et al.*, 2002). The ability to direct such events is extremely useful for both studying developmental changes and also for use in cell therapy (see Chapter 12).

9.   Adult stem cells

These are undifferentiated cells found among differentiated cells in a tissue or organ. Normally these cells can differentiate along a more limited pathway than embryonic stem cells to produce cells associated with the tissue. The cells serve to replace cells or repair tissue damage. Under certain conditions these cells may be induced into cell types other than those associated with the tissue from which they were derived. This is known as transdifferentiation or plasticity and is presently an active area of research.

Stem cells found in the bone marrow differentiate through the hematopoietic pathway to provide the extensive range of mature cell types. The hematopoietic stem cells are important for the continuous replacement of the cells found in the blood system. The hematopoietic pathway involves differentiation of cells through four stages – stem cells, early progenitor cells, progenitor cells and mature cells. The two distinct progenitor lineages (lymphoid and myeloid lineage) are shown in *Figure 2.7*. The lymphoid progenitor cells produce the mature T-lymphocytes, B-lymphocytes and natural killer cells from progenitor cells that are stimulated to differentiate by various interleukins (IL-2, IL-3, IL-6, IL-7). The myeloid lineage forms erythroid cells that can differentiate into monocytes, macrophages, neutrophils, eosinophils, basophils, megakaryocytes and erythrocytes. The formation of erythrocytes is stimulated by the glycoprotein, erythropoietin, the production of which occurs in the kidney and is enhanced by low oxygen levels (hypoxia). The steps of hematopoiesis are controlled by the microenvironment of the cells and secreted proteins (cytokines) from neighboring cells (stromal cells) promote the differentiation process *in vivo*. Isolated progenitor cells can also be expanded outside the body (*ex vivo*). The early-stage hematopoietic progenitor cells are characterized by a surface antigen called CD34 by which the cells can be isolated (Zandstra *et al.*, 1997). The most effective way of promoting the differentiation of these early progenitor hematopoietic cells in culture (*ex vivo*) is by cocultivation with stromal cells. Alternatively, conditioned stromal cell media or the addition of specific cocktails of recombinant allows expansion of the hematopoietic lineage. The use of a chemically defined medium containing recombinant cytokines is also the preferred method for therapeutic use because it ensures consistency and the absence of infectious agents. Many culture parameters affect the differentiation process including pH, osmolarity, temperature and media composition. The process has several therapeutic applications which are described in Chapter 12.

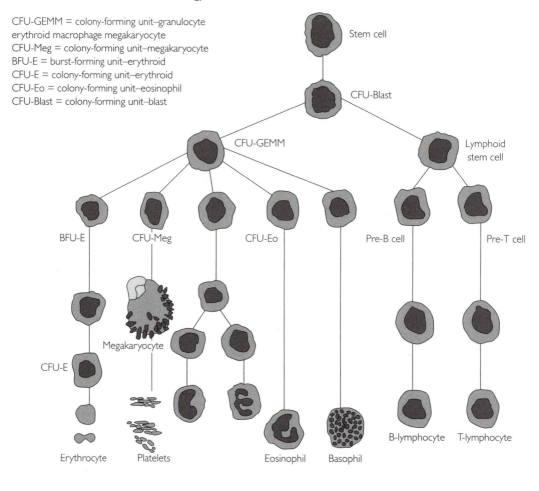

CFU-GEMM = colony-forming unit–granulocyte
erythroid macrophage megakaryocyte
CFU-Meg = colony-forming unit–megakaryocyte
BFU-E = burst-forming unit–erythroid
CFU-E = colony-forming unit–erythroid
CFU-Eo = colony-forming unit–eosinophil
CFU-Blast = colony-forming unit–blast

Figure 2.7

Differentiation of cells of the hematopoietic system. Modified from Inoue, et al., *1995.*

10. Transformed cells

Transformation has two different meanings in cell biology:

■   expression of foreign genes in bacteria;
■   change of animal cells from normal to infinite growth capacity.

In this section we are using the second definition. 'Normal' animal cells have a finite growth capacity but some cells acquire a capacity for infinite growth and such a population can be called an 'established' or 'continuous' cell line. This requires cells to go through a process called transformation, which causes the cells to lose their sensitivity to the stimuli associated with growth control.

Transformed cells may also lose their anchorage-dependence and often show some chromosome fragmentation. This genetic state is referred to as aneuploidy, which means that there is a slight alteration from the normal diploid state. The transformed cells have a high capacity for growth in relatively simple growth medium and without the need for growth factors.

Carcinogenesis *in vivo* is analogous, but not identical to the transformation of cells *in vitro*. Not all transformed cells are malignant, a characteristic defined by the ability to form tumors in animals. However, all tumor-derived cells grow continuously in culture. Examples include HeLa cells, which are derived from a cervical cancer (Gey *et al.*, 1952) and Namalwa cells, which derive from a human lymphoma. These cells are relatively easy to grow. They are robust and show good growth characteristics, which include a short doubling time and a low requirement for growth factors.

Cells can be transformed or 'immortalized' by a variety of techniques. This includes treatment with mutagens, viruses or oncogenes (Casalbore *et al.*, 1987).

An oncogene is defined as a gene that induces the formation of tumorigenic cells. The first 'tumor' virus to be recognized was Rous sarcoma virus which is a chicken retrovirus described by Rous in 1911. The viral oncogenes (e.g. v-myc) are derived from cellular genes – the proto-oncogenes (e.g.: c-myc).

Infection by retroviruses is a particularly effective method of immortalizing cells. These retroviruses express activated oncogenes (e.g. *myc* and *ras*), which cause cell transformation. The retroviruses are also useful for incorporating recombinant DNA into animal cells (see Chapter 6). Alternatively, some cells can transform spontaneously in culture. This has been observed particularly with rodent cells and may be explained by the tendency of such cells to harbor endogenous viruses.

11. Cells from a culture collection

For many applications, cell lines may be obtained from cell culture collections ('cell banks'), which have a large selection of well-characterized cell lines. This is far easier than having to rely on primary animal tissue for establishing cultures. Samples of cell suspensions ($\sim 10^7$ cells/ml) are offered for sale by the cell collections in frozen vials that can be transported in dry ice. On arrival the cells should be thawed and inoculated immediately into culture media or stored in liquid nitrogen.

Table 2.1 lists a few examples of commonly used cell lines which can be obtained from the major international culture collections. All these cells grow well in culture when provided with an appropriate growth medium. The full history of each cell line is available from the collection catalogs as well as a list of references indicating previous use of the cells.

The largest and most well-known international animal cell culture collections are given below. These collections contain well over 3000 well-characterized cell lines.

- The American Type Culture Collection (ATCC), 12301 Parklawn Drive, Rockville, Maryland 20852, USA: website: www.atcc.org.
- The European Collection of Animal Cell Culture (ECACC), Public Health Laboratory Service (PHLS), Centre for Applied Microbiology Research (CAMR), Porton Down, Salisbury SP4 OJG, UK: website: www.ecacc.org.

Table 2.1. Examples of common cell lines obtainable from culture collections

Cell line	Origin	Cell type	Comment
BHK	Baby hamster kidney	Fibroblast	Cells are anchorage-dependent but can be induced into suspension; used for vaccine production
CHO	Chinese hamster ovary	Epithelial	Cells will attach to a surface if available but will also grow in suspension; used extensively for genetic engineering
HeLa	Human cervical carcinoma	Epithelial	Fast-growing human cancer cell isolated in the 1950s
L	Mouse connective tissue	Fibroblast	Many culture techniques developed from the 1950s were based on this tumor cell line
L6	Rat skeletal muscle	Myoblast	Can be used to demonstrate the differentiation of a muscle cell
MDCK	(Madin Darby) canine kidney	Epithelial	Anchorage-dependent cells with good growth characteristics; used for veterinary vaccine production
MRC-5	Human embryonic lung	Fibroblast	Finite lifespan, 'normal' cells; used for human vaccine production
MPC-11	Mouse myeloma	Lymphoblast	Derived from a mouse tumor; secretes immunoglobulin
Namalwa	Human lymphoma	Lymphoblast	Derived from cells from a human suffering from Burkitt's lymphoma; used for alpha-interferon production
NB41A3	Mouse neuroblastoma	Neuronal	Tumor cells with good growth rate. Cells have nerve cell characteristics including a response to nerve growth factor
3T3	Mouse connective tissue	Fibroblast	Vigorous growth in suspension; cells used widely in the development of cell culture techniques
WI-38	Human embryonic lung	Fibroblast	Finite lifespan, 'normal' cells; used for human vaccine production
Vero	African green monkey kidney	Fibroblast	An established cell line capable of continuous growth but with many 'normal' diploid characteristics; used for human vaccine production

Other services offered by these establishments are:

■ the safe storage of private cell lines. This is useful for the maintenance of a master stock of important cells;

■ tests for contamination in cell lines;

■ characterization of cell lines. This includes isoenzyme analysis, karyotyping and DNA fingerprinting (see Chapter 5).

References

Casalbore, P., Agostini, E. and Alema, S. (1987) The v-myc oncogene is sufficient to induce growth transformation of chick neuroretina cells. *Nature* **326**: 188–190.

Gey, G.O., Coffman, W.D. and Kubicek, M.T. (1952) Tissue culture studies of the proliferative capacity of cervical carcinoma and normal epithelium. *Cancer Res.* **12**: 364–365.

Inoue, N., Takeuchi, M., Ohashi, H. and Suzuki, T. (1995) The production of recombinant human erythropoietin. *Biotechnology Annual Review* **1**: 297–313.

Sykes, J.A., Whitescarver, J., Briggs, L. and Anson, J.H. (1970) Separation of tumor cells from fibroblasts with use of discontinuous density gradients. *J. Natl. Cancer Inst.* **44**: 855–864.

Thomson, J.A., Itskovitz-Eldor, J., Shapiro, S.S. *et al.* (1998) Embryonic stem cell lines derived from human blastocytes. *Science* **282**: 1145–1147.

Wichterle, H., Lieberam, I. and Porter, J.A. (2002) Directed differentiation of embryonic stem cells into motor neurons. *Cell* **110**: 385–397.

Zandstra, P.W., Conneally, E., Petzer, A.L., Piret, J.M. and Eaves, C.J. (1997) Cytokine manipulation of primitive human hematopoietic cell self-renewal. *Proc. Natl Acad. Sci. (USA)* **94**: 4698–4703.

Further reading

The experimental procedures for the disaggregation of tissue and establishing a primary culture are well described in Chapter 9 of:

Freshney, R.I. (2000) *Culture of Animal Cells: A manual of basic technique*, 4th Edn. A.R. Liss, New York.

An account of the expansion of cells in the hematopoietic lineage is given in:

McAdams, T.A., Miller, W.M. and Papoutsakis, E.T. (1996) Hematopoietic cell culture therapies (Part 1): cell culture considerations. *Trends Biotechnol.* **14**: 341–349.

The following are two accounts of the procedures for handling cells in culture collections written by the collection organizers at the ATCC and ECACC.

Doyle, A., Hay, R. and Kirsop, B.E. (1990) *Living Resources for Biotechnology: Animal Cells*. Cambridge University Press, Cambridge.

Hay, R.J. (1986) Preservation and characterisation. In: Freshney, R.I. (ed.) *Animal Cell Culture: A Practical Approach*, pp.71–112. IRL Press, Oxford.

A description of the potential for stem cell technology is given in:

Smith, A.G. (2001) Embryo-derived stem cells: of mice and men. *Annu. Rev. Cell Dev. Biol.* **17**: 435–462.

Protocol 2.1

Preparing a primary cell culture of chick embryo fibroblasts

Equipment

Laminar flow cabinet

Forceps

Screen cup + 220 μm mesh (Sigma)

Materials

10 embryonated eggs

Hank's balanced salt solution (calcium- and magnesium-free)

Glass beads (1 mm diameter; Sigma)

0.2% (v/v) trypsin (1:1250) in Hank's balanced salt solution

Dulbecco's modification of Eagle's medium (DMEM)

Fetal calf serum (FCS)

Phosphate buffered saline (PBS)

Protocol

1. Clean 10 fertile 10-day-old incubated eggs with 70% ethanol.

2. Open the broad end of each egg with sterile scissors and carefully remove a piece of shell with the white membrane underneath.

3. Remove the embryos by sterile forceps, discard each head and transfer the trunk to a Petri dish containing 10 ml of sterile Hank's balanced salt solution (Ca- and Mg-free).

4. Wash ×2 with the salt solution to remove erythrocytes.

5. Remove and discard the internal organs with forceps.

6. Wash the remaining carcass ×3 with salt solution.

7. Transfer to a dry sterile tissue culture dish and chop into small pieces with sterile scissors.

8. Transfer to a flask containing 0.5 g glass beads (1 mm diameter) suspended in 1 ml PBS.

9. Add 20 ml 0.2% (v/v) trypsin (1:1250) in Hank's balanced salt solution and swirl the flask gently for 30 seconds.

10. Allow the larger fragments to sediment, then remove and discard the supernatant containing the erythrocytes.

11. Add a further 20 ml of trypsin, agitate for 30 seconds and transfer supernatant to a sterile centrifuge tube. Repeat this trypsin extraction ×5.

12. Centrifuge the tube at 300 **g** for 5 min to pellet the cells. Re-suspend in Hank's balanced salt solution containing 5% fetal calf serum.

13. Pour the cell suspension through a sterile 220 μm mesh screen cup to remove all debris.

14. Pellet the cells from the suspension and re-suspend in growth medium (DMEM + 10% FCS).

Notes

This entire procedure should be carried out in a laminar flow cabinet under sterile conditions. The process combines proteolytic digestion with mechanical agitation to cause individual cells to disperse into a liquid suspension. The addition of a serum-supplemented medium after trypsinization is important to inhibit further activity of the trypsin. Digestion of the tissue may be aided by the proteolytic enzyme collagenase and by the addition of chelating agents such as Versene or ethylene-diaminetetraacetic acid (EDTA).

Protocol 2.2

Isolation of lymphocytes from a blood sample

Materials

Diluted blood: Add an equal volume of balanced salt solution to anticoagulant-treated blood

Balanced salt solution (120 mM NaCl, 0.55 mM glucose, 5 μM CaCl$_2$.2H$_2$O, 0.98 μM MgCl$_2$.6H$_2$O, 0.54 mM KCl, 14.5 mM Tris)

Protocol

1. Add 3 ml Ficoll-Paque to a centrifuge tube.

2. Layer 4 ml of diluted blood sample on to the Ficoll-Paque.

3. Centrifuge at 400 *g* for 30 minutes at room temperature.

4. Remove the upper layer (plasma) with a Pasteur pipette, leaving the lymphocyte layer undisturbed.

5. Transfer the lymphocyte layer into another centrifuge tube using a minimal volume.

6. Add three volumes of balanced salt solution.

7. Aspirate with a pipette to ensure adequate suspension of the cells in the liquid.

8. Centrifuge at 100 *g* for 10 min and discard the supernatant.

9. Re-suspend the cell pellet and repeat steps 6 to 8 above.

Notes

The upper layer following the initial centrifugation contains blood plasma and is a good source of platelets. Washing the lymphocytes in salt solution ensures removal of the platelets. Granulocytes and erythrocytes form the lower layer after centrifugation. Transferring a minimal volume of the lymphocyte band ensures minimal granulocyte contamination. Typically this procedure recovers up to 80% of the lymphocytes from the original blood sample.

Chapter 3

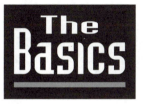

Basic equipment and laboratory design: what you need to get started in cell culture

1. Introduction

The purpose of this chapter is to review some of the basic requirements for setting up a small-scale culture laboratory for handling mammalian cell lines. This will include a description of a suitable laboratory environment in which to manipulate such cells and some of the basic laboratory equipment needed.

2. Laboratory design

A cell culture laboratory should allow the sterile handling of cultured cells with a minimal level of contamination. The growth rate of bacterial or fungal cells is usually so much greater than that of mammalian cells that no level of contamination can be tolerated in an animal cell culture. However, it is impractical to design a laboratory that is totally free of potentially contaminating microorganisms. The laboratory is generally designed to minimize the risk of contamination for an experienced worker. Thus, the maintenance of noncontaminated cultures is as much a product of good experimental technique as a clean germ-free environment.

In the development of animal cell culture techniques during the 1920s and 30s, Alexis Carrel used methods borrowed from surgical practices employed in hospital operating rooms. This included full gowning with surgical dress in a sterile room. However, nowadays these methods would be regarded as rather extreme and are not normally considered necessary in a modern laboratory. To minimize the risks of contamination, several features can be incorporated into the designated 'clean' laboratory.

An important feature of the laboratory should be a good physical separation of the sterile handling area from the areas for wash-up and sterilization. Ideally these may be separated in different laboratories. Cell culture facilities are often located in small rooms where there is minimal traffic of personnel. A small room containing a standard class II laminar flow cabinet is ideal because the air flow through the sterile exhaust of the cabinet should maintain a low particle count in the environment. The laminar flow cabinet (hood), microscope and incubator should be positioned close together so that physical transfer of cultures will be minimized. When it is not possible to have an independent sterile handling laboratory, it is at least necessary to ensure that the sterile handling area of a larger laboratory is positioned in a region where there is minimal movement of people. The area used for non-sterile work such as the wash-up facility and disposal of used culture flasks should be positioned at the other side of the laboratory from the clean area. A typical plan for a cell culture laboratory is shown in *Figure 3.1*. This is a self-contained laboratory suitable for use by two or three people. In a larger facility it would be essential to include separate rooms for the clean area and wash-up area.

The incoming air into the laboratory may be filtered through a high-efficiency particulate air (HEPA) filter or electronic filter that may be incorporated into the ceiling space. The incoming air pressure may be increased to cause a slight positive pressure within the laboratory. Air cooling ('conditioning') may often be necessary because of the heat generated by the incubators and other electronic equipment in the laboratory. Such measures will reduce the level of potential airborne contaminants in the laboratory environment. Sterile handling of cultures is generally carried out in a laminar flow cabinet into which only the operator's arms enter the sterile work area. This reduces air currents and the potential for contamination carried by laboratory workers. This minimizes the potential of contaminants entering opened culture flasks. Other areas of the laboratory should be maintained clean by removal of unnecessary clutter and application of antiseptic cleaning agents at regular intervals.

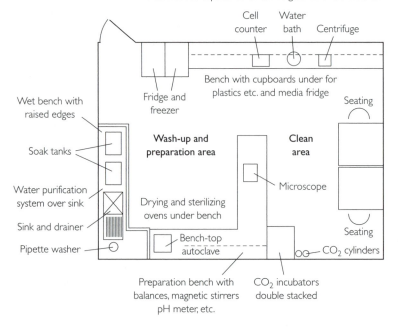

Figure 3.1

Plan for a cell culture laboratory (modified from Wigley, 1994).

3. Washing re-usable glassware

The general use of presterilized tissue culture-grade plasticware has meant a decrease in the amount of washing necessary in the average research laboratory involved in cell culture. It is difficult and time-consuming to wash glassware sufficiently so that it is free of potentially cytotoxic detergent to enable reproducibility in cell culture. The advantages of single-use plastic culture vessels include consistency in operation as well as a decreased preparation time. Nevertheless there is still a need for an adequate washing facility in most laboratories to prepare the spinner flasks, beakers and measuring cylinders that are used routinely. These all require a scrupulous washing regime prior to use or prior to sterilization. Any failure in the washing operation allows the possibility of the introduction of contaminants (e.g. traces of heavy metal) into the cultures and would likely result in a cytotoxic effect causing lowered cell growth or an altered metabolism.

It is necessary to soak all re-usable glassware in a hypochlorite solution (Chloros) as soon as possible after use. This will prevent the possibility of a build-up of dried protein residues that are difficult to remove. It is desirable to have access to a sink deep enough to accommodate all the dirty glassware at one time and to allow the complete immersion of the largest glass items. Generally a sink depth of around 45 cm is suitable. If the wash-up area is outside the culture laboratory then the glassware may be stored in a bucket next to the work area before removal to the main sink. Prior to immersion in the soak tank it is advisable to rinse glassware under a cold tap, remove any tape and remove any marker pen labeling with acetone. Soaking should be for several hours or preferably overnight.

In many laboratories a suitable washing machine (e.g. Lancer) is available for washing after the initial soaking. The desired procedure, either manually or by machine is to wash with a detergent and rinse with a dilute acid. Washing machine manufacturers have recommended conditions for this as appropriate for a particular machine. These procedures are followed by repeated sequential washes in tap water and then distilled or reverse-osmosis water.

The glassware should be dried in a hot air oven at around 100°C before use or sterilization (Roberts, 1994). Items that are not immediately sterilized should be kept covered or inverted on a clean surface until required.

Although individually packed presterilized plastic pipettes are available, many laboratories choose to re-use standard glass pipettes in cell culture operations. These may be washed and sterilized by following a similar procedure to that recommended for other glassware. Pipettes may be washed in a free-standing cylindrical pipette washer which is generally made of polypropylene. After removal of the cotton plug from each pipette, they should be placed tip uppermost into the cylinder container of the pipette washer for overnight soaking in a hypochlorite solution. This is then followed by 4–6 hours of washing using the siphon-type automatic washer. Initially this should be done with tap water and then with distilled or reverse-osmosis water. The pipettes are then dried in an oven before re-plugging with cotton wool and sorting pipettes of the same size into metal cans. These may be sterilized by dry heat (160°C for 1 hour).

4.   Biosafety/laminar flow cabinets

Sterile operations in a cell culture laboratory are normally undertaken in cabinets (commonly called 'hoods'), which serve the purpose of minimizing the chance of culture contamination and ensure the safety of the operator.

For media preparation, or when handling nonprimate cell lines, culture manipulations can be conducted in a small front-opening cabinet. The cabinets are relatively cheap and are equipped with an ultraviolet (UV) light source to prevent contamination of the cabinet surface when not in use but may not have an internal air flow. The surface of the cabinet should be disinfected regularly and bottles or flasks should not be stored in the cabinet. Good technique will ensure that cultures do not become contaminated. However, it must be noted that this system does not offer operator protection against possible pathogens (Harbour and Steffe, 1992).

If human or other primate cells are used then some protection is required against the possibility of transmission of infectious agents. For this purpose most cell culture laboratories have an open-fronted laminar flow cabinet in which only the operator's arms enter the sterile area. The cabinet offers a space containing a vertical flow of filtered air and a horizontal working surface that can be disinfected. The most commonly used cabinet for cell culture is 1.22 m long and designated as class II (*Figure 3.2*). The classification is a measure of the biological safety (Doyle and Allner, 1990).

A class II cabinet is suitable for work with low-to-moderate toxic or infectious agents. There is an inward flow of air drawn into the sterile working area of the cabinet through a high-efficiency particulate air (HEPA) filter. The direction of flow offers personnel protection. Most of the air (70–80%) is recirculated to form an air curtain which serves to maintain sterile space for culture manipulation. The air curtain formed in the internal front face of the cabinet has a typical flow rate of 0.4 m/s. The exhausted air is also forced through a HEPA filter and this serves to protect the surrounding environment from any potential pathogens or toxic compounds. The design of the class II cabinet is such that there is free access for the operator's hands but a Perspex cover prevents the operator breathing over the working surface. The HEPA filters are designed to trap extraneous airborne particles or aerosols. They are constructed from a continuous sheet of submicron glass fiber folded back and forth over a corrugated spacer as a support. The common HEPA filter in a class II cabinet ensures a 99.99% efficiency of entrapment of 0.3 μm particles. The cabinet should be located in a corner of the laboratory free from draughts and air movement. A source of UV light is an optional feature that can be built into these cabinets. The purpose of the UV light is to maintain sterility when the cabinet is not in use. It is also advisable to spray and wipe the horizontal working surface of the cabinet with 70% ethanol before use.

The class III cabinet is a totally enclosed system found in specialized laboratories designed to handle high-risk pathogens. This type of cabinet is completely sealed and contains glove pockets to allow manipulation of the cultures. The exhausted air from the cabinet is filtered through at least two HEPA filters to ensure the complete removal of all pathogens. All equipment entering the cabinet is passed through an air lock and removed directly into an autoclave. The class III cabinets are required for handling highly patho-

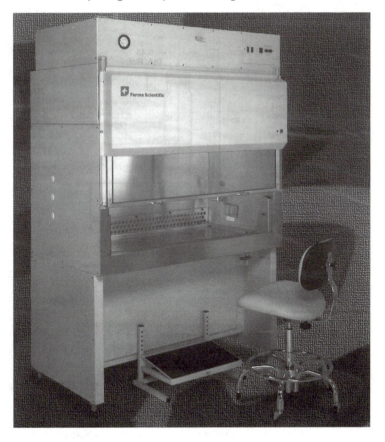

Figure 3.2

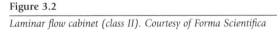

Laminar flow cabinet (class II). Courtesy of Forma Scientifica

genic material such as virus-producing human cell lines or tissue samples carrying known human pathogens.

5. Incubators

Incubators are a basic necessity for maintaining a constant temperature during cell culture, usually at 37°C for mammalian cells. These incubators may range from temperature-regulated boxes to more elaborate systems that can control temperature, humidity and CO_2 (*Figure 3.3*). These three parameters are essential for maintaining the consistency of culture conditions as well as preserving the viability of the cells. A slight decrease in temperature from the optimal may slow the cell growth rate but an increase in temperature is likely to be far more detrimental to the cells. Cells will survive at 39°C only for a few hours and they will die rapidly at a temperature above 40°C. Maintenance of a humidified atmosphere is essential to prevent loss of medium by evaporation in nonsealed culture systems such as Petri dishes and multi-well plates or in T-flasks without an airtight cap.

An enriched CO_2 atmosphere of the incubator chamber is usually maintained as a buffering system, which involves an equilibration with the bicarbonate contained in the culture medium. The required level of CO_2 to

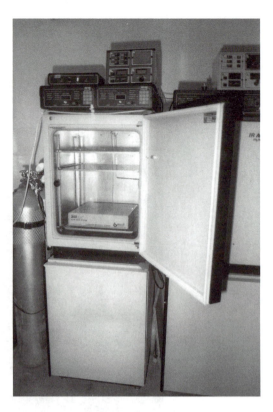

Figure 3.3

Double chamber CO$_2$ incubator. Courtesy of Forma Scientifica

maintain a culture pH at around 6.9–7.4 will depend upon the bicarbonate concentration of the medium (*Table 3.1*). Most growth media are rated for either 5% or 10% CO$_2$ and this necessitates a constant supply of CO$_2$ into the incubation chamber.

Abnormal CO$_2$ levels in the incubator are reflected by a change in pH of the culture medium as observed by the color. Too low a level of CO$_2$ causes an increase in culture pH whereas too high a level of CO$_2$ causes a decrease in pH. The CO$_2$ level can be monitored by a Fyrite test kit. In this simple apparatus a gas sample is pumped manually into an absorbing liquid by a rubber bulb. The level the liquid rises in the glass column indicates the % CO$_2$.

Table 3.1. Recommended levels of CO$_2$ in incubators with different media

Bicarbonate in medium (mM)	Recommended CO$_2$ level in gas phase	Example of medium
4	Atmospheric	Hank's BSS
26	5%	RPMI 1640
44	10%	DMEM

The disadvantage of the bicarbonate–CO_2 buffer system is that cultures may become alkaline very quickly when removed from the incubator. It is also possible to use an organic buffer to maintain culture pH. HEPES (N-2-hydroxyethylpiperazine-N'-2-ethanesulfonic acid; pK_a = 7.3 at 37°C) or MOPS (morpholinopropane sulfonic acid; pK_a = 7.0 at 37°C) at a concentration of 10–20 mM will maintain culture pH without an enriched CO_2 atmosphere. In the presence of HEPES the CO_2 level can be reduced to around 2% with a concomitant decrease in bicarbonate concentration. The organic buffers may be used in addition to the bicarbonate–CO_2 buffering system when a high degree of pH control is required. The disadvantage of using organic buffers is that the medium becomes expensive and therefore they are not generally used for routine culture.

The CO_2 incubator in which a fixed CO_2 tension is maintained in a humidified atmosphere has now become a standard piece of equipment in a cell culture laboratory. In a small laboratory the CO_2 cylinders are secured to a rack alongside the incubator. Gas is fed via a reducing valve on the cylinder head through pressure tubing to an intake port that passes through a filter before entering the incubation chamber. For older designed CO_2 incubators there is a constant flow of a CO_2/air mixture with each gas supplied separately from a different cylinder and mixed to set proportions via gas burettes. This has the disadvantage of excessive usage of CO_2 and if the CO_2 supply runs out then the constant air flow flushes out any remaining CO_2 from the incubator.

In a modern system two CO_2 cylinders are mounted alongside each incubator. Each cylinder has two regulator valves. One is a high-pressure gauge that measures the pressure in the cylinder with a range of 0–2000 psi and a second is a low-pressure gauge (0–30 psi) measuring the gas pressure into the incubator. Pressure tubing connects the low-pressure gauges of the two cylinders to a switching device, which if automated will switch the CO_2 supply from cylinder one to cylinder two if the pressure falls below a certain level (typically 4 psi). This automated switchover unit is essential to ensure a constant CO_2 supply (*Figure 3.4*).

The % CO_2 in the incubation chamber is controlled by a valve governed by intermittent readings of an infrared gas analyzer. Such a sensor system is built into the control box of the incubator and is capable of maintaining a constant CO_2 level to an accuracy of ±0.1%. The infrared controller measures the CO_2 level independently of humidity and incorporates a correction for temperature.

Air is normally pumped into the incubation chamber by a small pump via a filter. The circulation of air ensures an even temperature throughout the chamber. The chamber temperature is effectively controlled by a large jacket through which the circulation of water can ensure a uniform temperature of ±0.2°C. Other temperature control devices can be used but traditionally they have been assumed to be not as good as water jackets in ensuring an even chamber temperature. However, modern direct heat CO_2 incubators are available with heating elements on all sides of the outer chamber wall. Microprocessor control can ensure thermal stability in these incubators at least as well as in the water-jacketed type. The main advantage of the direct heat incubators is that they are considerably lighter than the water-jacketed type.

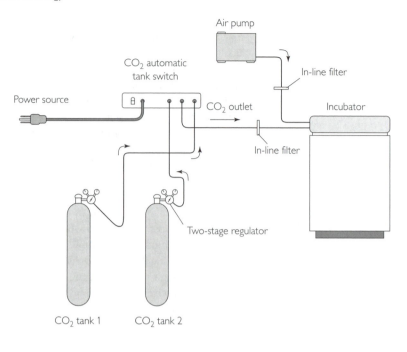

Figure 3.4

A typical gas control system for a modern CO_2 incubator.

The inner volume of a CO_2 incubator is typically 60–220 liters. The inner chamber of the incubator is normally sealed by a glass door and in order to prevent excessive condensation on the glass, a source of radiant heat is provided in the outer door. A water tray in the bottom of the incubator over which air is circulated maintains the humidity. This prevents excessive evaporation from the culture vessels. It is important to prevent microbial growth in this water reservoir by the addition of a low concentration of a disinfectant detergent. Routine maintenance requires regular cleaning and disinfection of the inner walls and trays of the chamber, which are made of stainless steel. In some incubator models (e.g. Cytoperm from Heraeus) an automated disinfection routine involves the introduction of hot air at 180°C. For many laboratories double cabinet incubators are useful. One chamber is stacked above the other but they are independently regulated.

Figure 3.3 shows two incubator chambers stacked one on top of the other. The CO_2 is supplied from the cylinder seen on the left. The inner chamber of the incubator contains a series of racks onto which culture vessels can be placed.

6. Laboratory-scale culture flasks

In the past, culture flasks were made of borosilicate glass. The most common was the Roux bottle consisting of two flat sides with a typical surface area of 230 cm^2 per side for the attachment and growth of anchorage-dependent cells and a capacity for a 500 ml culture volume. The flasks were re-cycled and required washing and autoclaving before use – a process that could give rise to contamination. However, presterilized plastic flasks suitable for cell culture are now commercially available and are used by most laboratories. The plastic is polystyrene, which is treated to produce a surface amenable for cell attachment and growth. The tissue-grade plastic flasks are sterilized by gamma irradiation and are suitable for single use. The use of presterilized and disposable plastic flasks has significantly reduced any contamination arising from the culture vessels. There is no need for an extensive washing process, which is critical to ensure the complete removal of cytotoxic contaminants from glass containers.

Whatever material is used, the surface charge density is critical for the attachment of cells. Thus, the physical and chemical treatment of surfaces has a considerable effect on cell adhesion. New borosilicate glass flasks or bottles often show poor cell adherence but this can be improved by washing, sterilization and chemical treatment. An appropriate charge can be placed on the glass by alkali treatment. Typically, this involves addition of 0.1 M EDTA in 25 mM NaOH at 122°C for 30 minutes followed by washing with sodium carbonate. The negative charge on the surface of glass can be manipulated by the extent of alkali treatment. The effect of alkali treatment is to rupture the Si–O–Si bonds of the silica network forming SiO^- residues with counter ions of Na^+ on the surface structure. The depth of penetration of Na^+ depends on the extent of treatment. The state of the surface can be quantitatively assessed by the extent of adsorption of the positively charged quaternary ammonium dye, crystal violet. Cell attachment can be improved by increasing the negative charge to a level specific for each cell type.

The attachment of the negatively charged cell surface to a negatively charged substratum requires the presence of a divalent cation such as Ca^{2+} and Mg^{2+} in the culture medium. Electron microscopic analysis of the cell-surface interface shows the presence of a 50 Å protein layer between the cells and the substratum. This may originate from surface-active proteins secreted by the cells or from a serum supplement in the growth medium (Grinnell, 1978).

The polystyrene used to make most domestic plastic containers is unsuitable as a surface for cell attachment because it is hydrophobic and has no charge. The 'tissue culture-grade' plasticware available from commercial sources is generally made of polystyrene, which is treated to allow a negative surface charge (Maroudas, 1977). This provides a surface chemistry that is hydrophilic, wetable and negatively charged. The charge may be provided by short exposure of the polystyrene to sulfuric acid to allow sulfonation of the surface. Alternatively, the usual commercial process is corona-oxidation in which the plastic is exposed to a high-voltage electric arc. This also leads to a surface with a layer of negatively charged groups. The structure of the chemically modified polystyrene is shown in *Figure 3.5*. There has been shown to be an optimal surface charge for cell attachment at a negative charge density of 2–10 × 10^{14} charges per cm^2. The polystyrene growth surface may be further modified by applying a variety of anionic and cationic groups, as shown in *Figure 3.5*. The polymeric surface with both amine and carboxyl groups shown in *Figure 3.5* is available in sterilized culture flasks as Primaria products (Falcon). These surfaces are optimal for the growth of certain specialized cell lines.

Cells have also shown an ability to attach to various positively charged polymers. These include DEAE-dextran, polyacrylamide, polylysine, polyornithine,

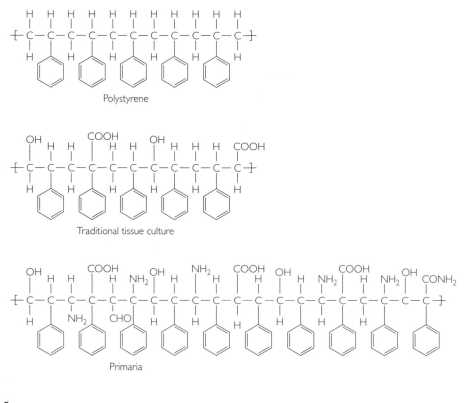

Figure 3.5

Modification of polystyrene to obtain a charged surface.

polyarginine, polyhistidine and protamine (McKeehan *et al.*, 1981). Thus, although the charge density on the surface appears to be a critical parameter, the charge may be positive or negative. Poly-D-lysine of molecular weight in the range 30–300 kDa or 30 000–300 000 Da has been used extensively as coating polymer for certain applications to provide a positive charge on glass or plastic (McKeehan and Ham, 1976). Washing a flask with a polylysine solution (10 μg/ml) is generally sufficient to apply the polymer coating. This may be useful to encourage the attachment of cells that usually grow in suspension. The surface charge density can also be manipulated by choosing a selected molecular weight of the polymer.

The choice of culture vessel for the growth of cells is dependent on the scale of operation and whether suspension or anchorage-dependent cells are required. Culture volumes from 10 μl to 10 000 liters are possible with existing commercially designed equipment. The smaller volume vessels (*Table 3.2*) are generally not equipped with control devices and it is accepted that pH and oxygen concentrations in culture may fluctuate during cell growth. However, the advantages of these vessels are that they can be handled in replicates and they are suitable for insertion into CO_2-enriched incubators. Most of these vessels offer a flat surface for cell attachment, although cells may be grown in suspension or surface-attached.

Table 3.2. Typical culture vessels suitable for cell growth

Culture vessel	Number of culture wells/unit	Maximum culture volume (ml)	Vessel size	Growth surface (cm^2)	Material
Multi-well plate	96	0.37	10.8 × 6.4 mm (D × diam.)	0.32	Plastic
Multi-well plate	24	3.4	17.6 × 15.5 mm (D × diam.)	1.88	Plastic
Multi-well plate	12	6.9	17.6 × 22.1 mm (D × diam.)	3.8	Plastic
Multi-well plate	6	16.8	17.6 × 34.6 mm (D × diam.)	9.4	Plastic
Medical flat bottle		10	125 ml	22	Glass
Medical flat bottle		15	250 ml	30	Glass
Roux bottle		50	500 ml	200	Glass
T-flask, 25		5.0	50 ml	25	Plastic
T-flask, 75		15–30	250 ml	75	Plastic
T-flask, 150		75	600 ml	150	Plastic
T-flask, 175		50–100	750 ml	175	Plastic
Roller bottle		100–200	1250 ml	490	Plastic
Roller bottle		100–250	2200 ml	850	Plastic
Roller bottle		100–500	4900 ml	1750	Plastic
Spinner flask		100	250 ml		Glass
Spinner flask		250	500 ml		Glass
Spinner flask		500	1000 ml		Glass
Spinner flask		1000	2000 ml		Glass
Cell factory, Nunc		1800		6000	Plastic

D, depth; diam., diameter

The most popular forms of plastic culture containers are multi-well plates, Petri dishes and flasks (usually referred to as Tissue culture flasks or T-flasks) made of tissue culture-grade polystyrene (*Figure 3.6*). The multi-well plates can accommodate many replicates of small-volume cultures (*Figure 3.7*). The 24-well plates hold 3 ml per well and are well suited for cell growth experiments, for example to test for toxicity or stimulatory activity (*Figure 3.7*). The 96-well plates hold a volume of 0.3 ml per well and are suitable for cloning or replicate assays. Rapid dispensing of solutions into the 96-well plate is made easy by use of a multi-well pipettor such as the one shown in *Figure 3.8*. These are lightweight and normally have an adjustable volume setting. The pipettors are designed for use with sterile pipette tips. The 96-well plate reader can be used to obtain simultaneous optical density data from all the wells from a single plate (*Figure 3.9*).

For some applications porous inserts for multi-well plates are available. These have polycarbonate or polyethylene terephthalate membranes of various pore sizes (0.4–8 μm). Cells can grow over the membrane provided. This may be useful to study cell polarity as access is provided to the basolateral and apical sides of the cell layer.

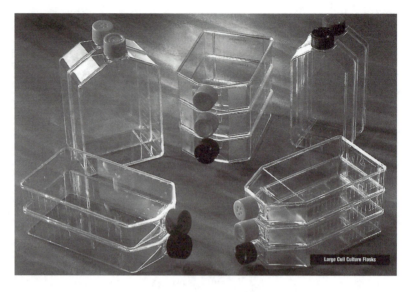

Figure 3.6

Tissue culture flasks (T-flasks). Courtesy of Corning Catalogue

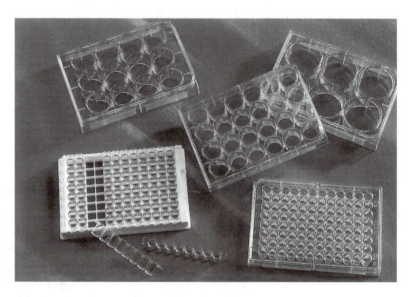

Figure 3.7

Multi-well plates.

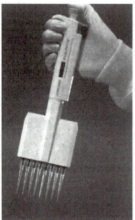

Figure 3.8

Multi-well pipettor.

The Petri dishes and T-flasks can accommodate cultures of 2–100 ml and are suitable for both anchorage-dependent and suspension cells. The T-flasks are designated by the surface area available for cell attachment. Thus T-25, T-75, T-150 and T-175 flasks have a growth area of 25–175 cm^2. A canted (angled) neck is provided so that sterile manipulation is easy. It is important to allow an equilibrium to develop between the gas phase of the flask and

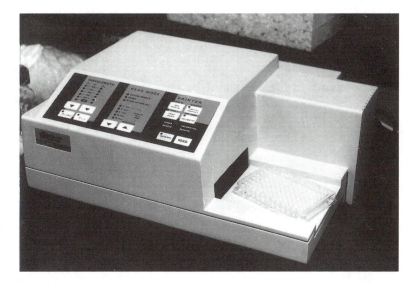

Figure 3.9

96-well plate reader.

the atmosphere of the incubator chamber. The T-flask caps can be adjusted to fit loosely, to allow gas exchange with the environment of the incubator. The caps should be closed tightly once the flasks are removed from the incubator. Some T-flasks have a ring of five holes in the plastic caps to allow gas exchange through an inner permeable membrane (lower right *Figure 3.6*).

Spinner bottles are straight-sided glass flasks containing a suspended central Teflon paddle containing a magnet, which turns and agitates the culture when placed on a magnetic stirrer (*Figure 3.10*). The stirring should be stable over a long period at a rotation speed of between 10 and 300 rpm. The bottle (or flask) is usually fitted with one or more side arms. These are useful for sampling or as ports for probes or tubing. Spinner bottles can be designed up to a capacity of 5–10 liters. Cultures above this volume require a top-driven motor for stirring. The spinner bottles are suited for growing suspension cells although they can be adapted for anchorage-dependent cells by the use of microcarriers. The spinner flasks are usually siliconized to prevent undue attachment of cells to the inner glass surface. This may be performed by application of dimethyldichlorosilane (Repelcote from Sigma).

An appropriately designed stirring base is required for operation of the spinner bottles. Most laboratory stirring bases used for chemical operations are unsuitable because they have poor speed control and cause excessive heating. The stirring bases used for cultures are required to maintain good speed control for long time periods and without excessive heating. The stirring bases are normally fitted with a tachometer for an accurate indication of the stirring rate. Although these cultures are often established in warm rooms many CO_2 incubators will also accommodate such a stirring base – the power line may be fitted through a sealable hole provided at the side of the incubator. However, prolonged use of stirring bases in a humidified

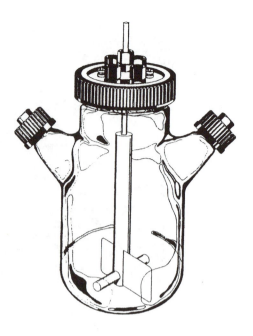

Figure 3.10

Spinner bottle with suspended paddle.

incubator can cause corrosion of the internal mechanical drives. This problem has been solved by some advanced stirrer modules (e.g. Bellco), which are sealed units placed inside the humidified incubator. A separate master controller that can control several stirrer modules is placed outside the incubator.

A larger surface area for cell growth is offered in roller bottles, which are cylindrical plastic containers that are placed on their side onto mechanical rollers (*Figure 3.11a*). The three standard sizes of roller bottles offer a growth surface of 490, 850 or 1750 cm² and can be filled with 250–500 ml of medium. The rolling mechanism allows the bottles to be rotated gently and the culture medium to flow continuously over the inner surface (*Figure 3.11b*). On inoculation into the culture medium, the cells attach and grow over the entire inner surface. The bottles are positioned to turn slowly along the long axis at between 5–60 revolutions per hour (rph). The volume of medium added should be just sufficient to provide a shallow covering of the cell monolayer. After each complete turn of a bottle the entire cell monolayer is transiently exposed to the medium. It is important to ensure that the rotation platform is perfectly horizontal otherwise cells at the high end of a flask will not be in contact with medium.

Roller bottle systems offer the possibility of high yields of anchorage-dependent cells in replicate cultures. They were originally developed for the large-scale culture of anchorage-dependent cells used in the commercial production of viral vaccines. Equipment is available to accommodate up to 30 000 bottles each of 1 liter capacity. However, the process is labor intensive as each roller bottle must be handled individually for media changes or cell harvest.

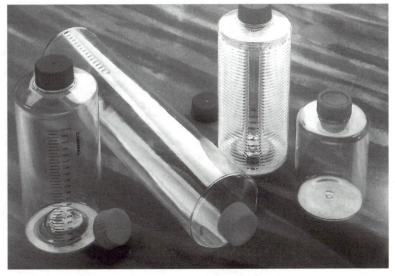

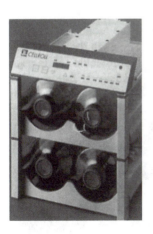

Figure 3.11b

Bottles in a roller system.

Figure 3.11a

Roller bottles of various sizes. Courtesy of Corning Catalogue

Microcarrier cultures offer an alternative means of producing large quantities of anchorage-dependent cells and these have now been adopted in most commercial processes for vaccine production (Chapter 12).

An alternative culture vessel for producing a large yield of cells on a laboratory scale is the multi-tray unit called the Cell Factory (Nunc). This is a plastic container that incorporates 10 large plastic trays sealed together. The total growth surface area is 6000 cm². No rolling is required and a maximum yield of over 10^9 anchorage-dependent cells can be expected. The system is designed for single use.

7. Microscopes

The two microscope types used for monitoring cells in culture are shown in *Figure 3.12*.

An inverted microscope is essential for examination of a cell culture at regular intervals to monitor the health and growth of cells (*Figure 3.12a*). The design of this microscope with the light source at the top and a long working distance condenser allows cells in flasks or even roller bottles to be viewed. Changes in the cell morphology, granularity and degree of spreading are all indicators that can be monitored by regular microscopic examination of cultures.

A standard microscope with a movable slide holder is required to count cells in a culture sample introduced into the counting chamber (*Figure 3.12b*). In addition to this, it is worthwhile inspecting culture samples under a microscope to determine if there are any significant changes to the appearance of the cells. Both types of microscope are essential for routine monitoring of cells in culture (Chapter 5).

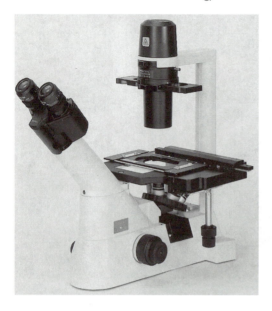

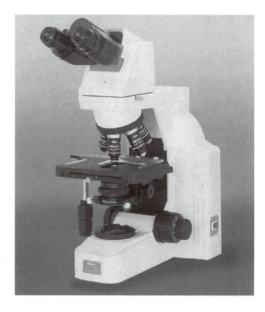

Figure 3.12a

Inverted microscope. Courtesy of Chay Keogh, on behalf of Nikon UK Ltd.

Figure 3.12b

Standard microscope. Courtesy of Chay Keogh, on behalf of Nikon UK Ltd.

8.   Centrifugation

A low-speed centrifuge is a requirement to harvest cells from culture (*Figure 3.13*). In general a centrifugal force of 150–200 g for 5–10 minutes should be sufficient to separate out cells from culture medium. Higher forces or longer times may cause damage to the cells by compacting them at the bottom of the centrifuge tube. Once centrifugation is completed, the supernatant should be decanted and the cells re-suspended. Typically swing-out buckets in a bench centrifuge will accommodate 50 ml or 15 ml plastic centrifuge tubes. The bucket size required will depend upon the volume of culture to be handled.

For reasons of safety the centrifuge rotor or individual buckets should be sealable to contain any spillage or breakage. Also, the centrifuge chamber should be sealed. Fine control of braking is desirable particularly if isolating cells from a concentration gradient. Gentle braking prevents disruption of the separated bands.

A benchtop microfuge may also be useful for higher-speed centrifugation of small volumes of reagents or media samples. These may develop precipitates after freezing. Also, many analytical techniques performed on cell culture media require precipitation of proteins prior to analysis.

9.   Liquid nitrogen storage

Cells can be stored for long periods at sub-zero temperatures. This permits cell stocks to be maintained in laboratories without having to resort to primary animal tissue. The maintenance of a cell stock guards against loss of

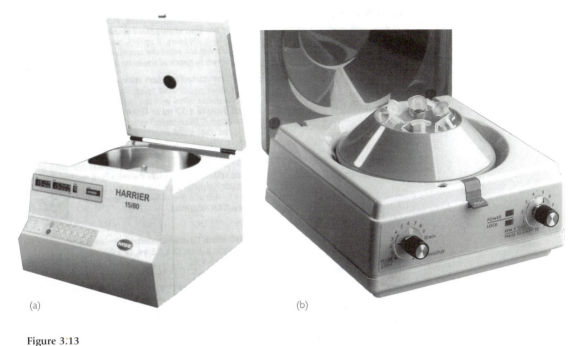

Figure 3.13

Low-speed laboratory centrifuges. (a) bench top, (b) microfuge. Courtesy of Sanyo Gallenkamp PLC.

a cell line by contamination or by genetic change. For cells that are grown continuously it is often desirable to store cells after various passages so that any genetic change can be monitored.

For a valuable cell line it is common to maintain a two-tiered cell bank – a master cell bank and a working cell bank. The master bank is a store of cells at early passage and established soon after receiving the original cells. The working bank is a store of cells formed by growth for several passages of one of the master bank samples. Future cell samples for inoculation of cultures are taken from the working cell bank and the master cell bank is accessed only when absolutely necessary. This practice is common in industrial production when the lifespan of the cell lines is carefully monitored.

Cells can be stored in a suspension (10^7 cells/ml) in a freezing medium that is dispensed into plastic ampoules (typically 2 ml). The freezing medium consists of growth medium or serum supplemented with a cryo-protectant such as 10% glycerol or dimethyl sulfoxide (DMSO) that will protect the cells from disruption during the freezing and thawing process. The cells are stable almost indefinitely in the cryo-protectant when held under liquid nitrogen ($-196°C$). Most cell culture laboratories will have liquid nitrogen storage canisters for such a purpose.

The method of freezing and thawing is important to maintain a high viability of the stored cells. Slow freezing and rapid thawing is recommended for maximum cell survival. The cell suspension can be frozen by placing the ampoules containing the cells in a polystyrene box held at $-70°C$ overnight. This ensures an initial freezing rate of about 1°C/min after which time the ampoules are placed directly into liquid nitrogen. Programable coolers are available to control the rate of cooling. These are based on a slow infusion of liquid nitrogen at a rate determined by the pre-set cooling program. However, they are not widely used in research laboratories because of the expense and the fact that there is no great advantage unless it is required to vary the rate of cell freezing. For recovering cells, the ampoules are transferred as quickly as possible from liquid nitrogen to a water bath at 37°C. The water bath should be covered for safety because there is a possibility that a damaged ampoule may explode if liquid nitrogen has penetrated the seal.

A liquid nitrogen freezer can range in capacity from 25–500 liters and may be narrow necked or wide necked. *Figure 3.14* shows typical laboratory cell storage units of different capacities. The freezers require regular addition of liquid nitrogen to maintain their temperature. The wide neck type of freezer has the advantage of easy access but the rate of liquid nitrogen evaporation is higher. The cells are stored in plastic vials (1–2 ml) which are lowered into liquid nitrogen for long-term storage. These are placed in large drawers (for wide-necked freezers) or attached to metal canes (for narrow-necked freezers). The cryogenic vials are contained in the plastic boxes (*Figure 3.15*), which are stacked in the metal racks before lowering into the liquid nitrogen. Depending on the size of the freezer, the storage capacity will vary between 250–15 000 plastic vials (or ampoules). A capacity for 1200–1500 vials is more than adequate for most research laboratories. Cryogenic plastic vials have strong seals to prevent leakage that could result from large temperature fluctuations. The liquid nitrogen reservoir needs to be replenished at regular intervals. This requires consistent and regular monitoring of the liquid nitrogen content in the reservoir, so that the stored vials of cells are maintained frozen. This may be performed with a dipstick. However, many modern freezers are fitted with an automatic indicator with an alarm, which sounds if the liquid nitrogen level gets too low. This lowers

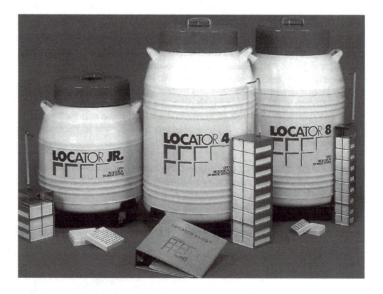

Figure 3.14

Liquid nitrogen storage facilities. Courtesy of Barnstead International

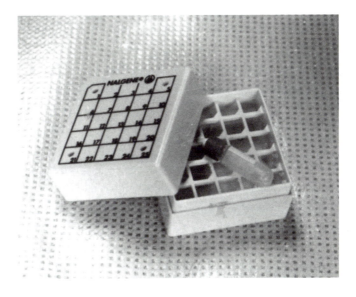

Figure 3.15

A cryogenic vial in a storage box.

the risk of damaging important cell stocks by inadvertently allowing the liquid nitrogen level to drop too low.

10. Osmometer

An important parameter of cell culture medium is the osmotic pressure expressed as osmolarity (number of particles per liter) or osmolality (number of particles per kilogram). Most measuring devices will determine the osmolality which approximates to the osmolarity in dilute solution. The effect of each component in the medium to the overall osmolarity is additive and dependent upon its dissociation. Therefore, 15 mM glucose will increase the osmolarity by 15 mOsm/l whereas 15 mM NaCl will increase the osmolarity by 30 mOsm/l.

The osmolarity of standard culture medium is approximately 300 mOsm/l and is optimal for most cell lines. Cells can normally tolerate variations within 10% of this value. However, care should be taken in adding supplements to the media as the osmolarity may be adversely affected.

The osmolarity of a culture may increase during cell growth as a result of the production of low-molecular-weight metabolites such as ammonia and lactic acid. An off-line measurement of the osmolarity of the culture may be made with a simple bench-top osmometer. The most common type is based on the measurement of the freezing point of the liquid. The principle is that the freezing point is lowered as the total number of all dissolved particles (ionic and nonionic) is increased. Water has a freezing point of 0°C whereas a saline solution with an osmolality of 1 Osmol/ kg has a freezing point of −1.858°C. Osmometers will measure the freezing point of a solution in comparison to that of water to an accuracy of ±0.001°C. Most models will measure within a range of 0–3000 mOsm/kg. Variations between different models of osmometers include the degree of automation for measuring multiple samples and the sample size required. In a micro-osmometer a sample size of 20–50 µl would be sufficient whereas sample sizes for a standard instrument are 0.2–2 ml.

References

Doyle, A. and Allner, K. (1990) Administration and safety. In: Doyle, A., Hay, R. and Kirsop, B.E. *et al.* (eds) *Living Resources for Biotechnology: Animal Cells*, pp. 50–62. Cambridge University Press, Cambridge.

Grinnell, F. (1978) Cellular adhesiveness and extracellular substrata. *Int. Rev. Cytol.* **53**: 65–144.

Harbour, C. and Steffe, R. (1992) Safety aspects of handling cells. In: Butler, M. and Dawson, M. (eds) *Cell Culture Labfax*, pp. 209–218. BIOS Scientific, Oxford.

Maroudas, N.G. (1977) Sulphonated polystyrene as an optimal substratum for the adhesion and spreading of mesenchymal cells in monovalent and divalent saline solutions. *J. Cell Physiol.* **90**: 511–519.

McKeehan, W.L. and Ham, R.G. (1976) Stimulation of clonal growth of normal fibroblasts with substrata coated with basic polymers. *J. Cell Biol.* **71**: 727–734.

McKeehan, W.L., McKeehan, K.A. and Ham, R.G. (1981) The use of low-temperature subculturing and culture surfaces coated with basic polymers to reduce the requirement for serum macromolecules. In: Waymouth, C., Ham, R.G. and Chapple, P.J. *et al.* (eds) *Requirements of Vertebrate Cells in vitro*, pp. 118–130. Cambridge University Press, Cambridge.

Roberts, P.L. (1994) Sterilization. In: Davis, J.M. (ed.) *Basic Cell Culture: A Practical Approach*, pp. 27–55. Oxford University Press, Oxford.

Wigley, C. (1994) The cell culture laboratory. In: Davis, J.M. (ed.) *Basic Cell Culture: A Practical Approach*, pp. 1–26. Oxford University Press, Oxford.

Further reading

Butler, M. (ed.) (1991) *Mammalian Cell Biotechnology: A Practical Approach.* Oxford University Press, Oxford.

Butler, M. (1996) *BASICS: Mammalian Cell Culture and Technology.* Oxford University Press, Oxford.

Butler, M. and Dawson, M.M. (eds) (1992) *Cell Culture: Labfax.* BIOS Scientific, Oxford.

Clynes, M. (ed.) (1998) *Animal Cell Culture Techniques.* Springer-Verlag, Berlin.

Davis, J.M. (ed.) (1994) *Basic Cell Culture: A Practical Approach.* Oxford University Press, Oxford.

Doyle, A. and Griffiths, J.B. (eds) (1998) *Cell and Tissue Culture: Laboratory Procedures in Biotechnology.* J. Wiley, New York.

Freshney, R.I. (2000) *Culture of Animal Cells: A Manual of Basic Technique*, 4th Edn. A.L. Liss, New York.

Jenkins, N. (ed.) (1999) *Animal Cell Biotechnology: Methods and Protocols.* Humana Press, New Jersey.

Morgan, S.J. and Darling, D.C. (1993) *Animal Cell Culture.* BIOS Scientific, Oxford.

Chapter 4

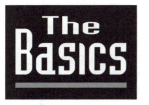

Growth and maintenance of cells in culture

This chapter considers some of the procedures for establishing cells in culture and the environment necessary to maintain favorable growth conditions.

1. How to culture cells and what to expect

1.1 Inoculation

Once cells are obtained from a culture collection or isolated from animal tissue, a culture can be initiated by inoculating the cells into sterile growth medium. In order to obtain a reasonable growth rate, cells should be inoculated at a density of 10^4–10^5 cells/ml. This will allow growth in a simple batch culture to around 10^6 cells/ml or to 10^5 cells/cm^2 on a solid surface in about 3–4 days. The increase in cell concentration in a culture can be expressed as the multiplication ratio, which is defined as C_f/C_i, where C_f is the final concentration and C_i the initial concentration. Expect a 10-fold increase in cell concentration in a simple batch culture.

Anchorage-dependent cells attach to an available growth surface within a few hours of inoculation. The attachment process involves the flattening and spreading of cells into a characteristic shape (Chapter 2).

Cell growth stops because of a nutrient limitation, an accumulation of a toxic metabolite or a lack of growth surface (for anchorage-dependent cells). If the medium is totally or partially replaced after 2 days, the maximum cell density may be higher.

1.2 Subculture

When cells stop growing in culture, new cultures can be established by inoculating some of the cells into fresh medium. This is called subculturing or passaging. It is important to subculture cells within a day or so of the maximum cell density to ensure continued growth in a new culture. Cells will lose their viability if they are left for too long before subculture. For cells grown in suspension, subculture involves dilution of the high-density culture with fresh medium. Dilutions from one in two to one in ten v/v would be suitable. It is advisable to pre-incubate growth medium in an incubator before inoculation. This ensures that the new culture is at the optimal temperature (37°C) and pH (~7.4) for maximum cell growth.

The subculture of anchorage-dependent cells involves detachment of the cells from the growth surface (substratum) of one culture flask and re-inoculation of the cells into fresh medium contained in a new culture flask. The cells are detached from their anchor by the process of trypsinization. Trypsinization was first introduced in the early days of cell culture (Rous and Jones, 1916) but was not fully developed until the 1950s when its use enabled the establishment of homogeneous cell populations.

A proteolytic enzyme such as trypsin will break down the proteins that bind the cells to the culture surface. The trypsin is added to washed cells in the culture flask for a short period that is long enough to dislodge the cells from the substratum but not too long to damage the cells. Cells will detach from a surface by treatment with trypsin for 15 minutes. It helps to bang the edge of the T-flask with your hand. Detachment of cells by trypsin is more efficient if magnesium and calcium ions are removed from the medium. This is achieved by combining trypsin with EDTA ('versene') administered in a Ca- and Mg-free salt solution. EDTA is a chelating agent that may be used alone for removal of weakly adherent cells. The action of trypsin is stopped by the addition of serum-supplemented medium and centrifugation to remove the cells. The excess protein present in the medium serves to reduce the trypsin activity. If the cells are grown in serum-free medium a soybean trypsin inhibitor can be used.

Cultures are given a passage number which indicates the number of sub-cultures performed since the cells were obtained or isolated. The relationship between the passage number and the generation number ('population doublings') depends upon the 'split ratio', which is the number of new cultures established at each stage of subculture. A typical cell population will double in one day.

The simplest case occurs where a confluent culture is sub-cultured into two new cultures i.e.: at a split ratio of 2. In this case, the generation number and the passage number are the same.

1.3   The phases of a culture

The culture will follow a growth pattern similar to that shown in *Figure 4.1*. Several phases of culture can be identified from this pattern.

The lag phase

This is an early phase in which there is no apparent increase in cell concentration. This phase is associated with the cellular synthesis of growth factors which may be required to reach a critical concentration before growth takes place. The length of this phase is dependent upon the culture medium formulation as well as the initial concentration and state of the cells. The lag phase tends to be longer at low inoculation densities or if the viability of the inoculated cells is low. This may occur if subculture is delayed. If a high density of cells with good viability is inoculated into the culture medium then the lag phase may be eliminated altogether. Transformed cells have a lower requirement for growth factors and often show no lag phase even when inoculated at lower concentrations.

In some circumstances, there may be a requirement to inoculate at a low cell density, for example during cell cloning. Cloning is the establishment of a culture from a single cell. This ensures that all cells in the culture are identical, i.e. a homogeneous population. In this situation cell growth can be enhanced by adding a feeder layer which consists of irradiated cells incapable of growth but metabolically active and capable of releasing growth factors into the medium.

The growth phase

During the exponential growth phase cells go through the cell cycle (see Chapter 5):

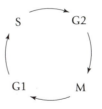

This phase involves an exponential increase in cell number which can be represented by the following equation:

$$N = N_o.2^X$$

or

$$\log_{10}N = \log_{10}N_o + X.\log_{10}2$$

where N = final cell concentration, N_o = initial cell concentration and X = number of generations of cell growth.

The number of generations (X) for a cell inoculum of 10^5 cells/ml which increases to a density of 10^6 cells/ml can be calculated as follows:

$$\log_{10}10^6 = \log_{10}10^5 + X.\log_{10}2$$

Therefore:

$$X = \frac{(\log_{10}10^6 - \log_{10}10^5)}{\log_{10}2} = \frac{1}{\log_{10}2} = 3.32 \text{ generations}$$

The doubling time during cell growth can be calculated from the equation:

$$t_D = \frac{T}{X}$$

where t_D = doubling time, T = total elapsed time and X = number of generations.

Thus, for a culture in which an initial cell density of 10^5 cells/ml reaches 10^6 cells/ml in 3 days the average doubling time is 0.904 days or 22 h.

Animal cells normally exhibit a doubling time of between 15–25 h during the exponential growth phase.

The specific growth rate (μ) is another growth parameter which is often calculated. This is a measure of the rate of increase of cell number (or biomass) at a certain cell concentration.

$$\mu = \frac{dN}{dt} \cdot \frac{1}{N}$$

or

$$\ln N = \ln N_o + \mu.t$$

where N_o = initial cell concentration, N = cell concentration at time and t = elapsed time from the start of cell growth.

The value of μ (h^{-1}) can be calculated from the slope of a plot of ln N against time, t. For the growth curve shown in *Figure 4.1* the specific growth

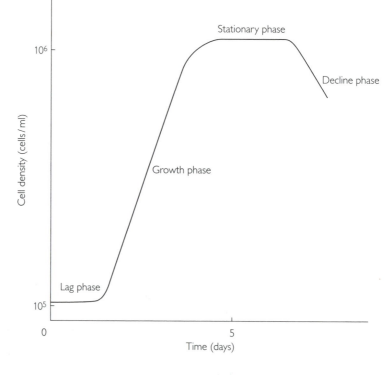

Figure 4.1

Cell growth in culture.

rate is 0.032 h^{-1}. There is also a simple relationship between the specific growth rate and doubling time.

If: $N = 2 \times N_o$, then $\ln 2 = \mu.t = \mu \times$ doubling time (t_D). Therefore:

$$\mu = \frac{\ln 2}{t_D} = \frac{0.6931}{t_D}$$

The stationary phase

This phase occurs when there is no further increase in cell concentration. During the stationary phase, death rate = growth rate.

At this point cell growth is limited by one of a number of conditions:

■ nutrients may have been depleted to a level that cannot support further cell growth;

■ the accumulation of metabolic by-products may have reached a level which is inhibitory to cell growth;

■ the cells may have formed a complete cover over the growth surface. Growth may stop when a single monolayer of cells covers the available substratum (called 'confluence'). This phenomenon is associated with cell–cell interaction (see Chapter 2).

During the stationary phase the cells may be metabolically active even though growth is not occurring. For example, in some cases high productivity of secreted proteins may occur during this phase.

The decline phase

This phase occurs as a result of cell death. Cell viability is lowest during the decline phase of culture – shown by a large difference between total and viable cell counts (see Chapter 5). The measured viable cell concentration decreases as the cells lyse and their intracellular metabolites are released into the growth medium. There are two possible mechanisms of cell death in culture – apoptosis or necrosis.

Apoptosis is a cell suicide mechanism observed to occur in culture or *in vivo* under normal physiological conditions (Cotter and Al-Rubeai, 1995). The process is characterized by a programmed pattern of cellular events. Apoptosis is a normal physiological mechanism of cell death. Abnormalities in the process have been implicated in tumorigenesis. During apoptosis endogenous endonucleases are activated to cleave the DNA into fragments of about 180 basepairs. The cell membrane assumes a characteristic ruffled appearance with many blebs. This is followed by cell shrinkage, nuclear condensation and fragmentation of the cell into discrete membrane-enclosed apoptotic bodies (*Figure 4.2*). *In vivo*, the apoptotic bodies generated by cell breakdown are phagocytosed by adjacent cells.

Apoptosis is thought to be important *in vivo* in regulating the proliferation of certain cell types for example, following immunological stimulation of lymphocytes.

In cell cultures apoptosis may be initiated by the depletion of nutrients. This causes the cells to go into a decline phase rapidly with a limited stationary phase. This is observed particularly with certain cell types for example, lymphocyte hybridomas (see Chapter 8).

The alternative mechanism of cell death is necrosis, which follows cellular injury. This does not involve the cell fragmentation characteristic of apoptosis and the loss of cell viability in culture is relatively slow. Necrosis is a passive process that normally occurs when cells are subject to sudden severe stress. This is characterized by a breakdown of the plasma membrane leading to cell swelling and eventual cell rupture.

2. The importance of aseptic techniques

The major cause of failure and frustration associated with the operation of cell cultures is the problem of contamination. Cultures are susceptible to

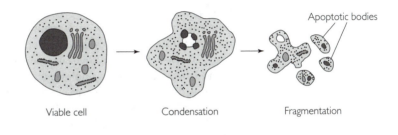

Viable cell   Condensation   Fragmentation

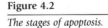

Figure 4.2

The stages of apoptosis.

overgrowth by bacteria because of the difference in growth rates. Typical doubling times are:

- animal cell = 24 h;
- bacteria = 30 min.

The slow growth rate of animal cells makes the culture particularly vulnerable to the fast growth rate of potential microbial contaminants such as bacteria and fungi. The safeguard against this problem is the meticulous use of standard aseptic microbiological techniques for all transfer operations.

2.1   How to prevent contamination

The aseptic techniques necessary for cell culture can now be performed easily in a well-designed laboratory and are far less elaborate than those originally conceived by Carrel (see Chapter 1). The major source of contamination is airborne and arises from inadequate aseptic techniques and most often originates from human contact such as from hands, breath or hair. Equipment and culture supplies are now available to minimize these risks of contamination (Chapter 3). The risks can also be reduced further by careful attention to detail when handling cultures. The following points are important to reduce this source of contamination.

- Wash hands with antiseptic soap before and after procedures involving handling cells. Latex gloves may be worn.
- Limit access to the laboratory when experiments are in progress.
- Decontaminate working surfaces before and after each procedure.
- Use a sterile space (e.g. laminar flow cabinet) for all manipulations.
- Ensure that there is a barrier between the operator's face and the culture. This could be a face mask or more usually the perspex front of a laminar flow cabinet.
- Use presterilized plastic culture flasks or ensure the adequacy of an in-house sterilization operation. The plastic culture flasks are only used once.
- Purchase media and serum from a reputable supplier to ensure contamination does not arise from this source. In the past, animal serum has been a source of mycoplasma infection but all batches of serum are now tested by the major suppliers and should be certified as mycoplasma-free. Mycoplasmas are Gram-negative bacteria (0.3–0.5 µm) capable of growth within the animal cell cytoplasm. This type of contamination is very difficult to detect in cell culture.

Media prepared in-house can be checked for sterility by incubation of a sample in a variety of broths or nutrient plates. Two commonly used isolation media suitable for revealing bacterial or fungal contamination are fluid thioglycollate medium and soybean-casein digest, both of which are available as dehydrated media. Samples can be inoculated into these media and contamination is revealed by increased turbidity. Incubation times for each sterility test should be at least 7 days.

The incorporation of antibiotics such as penicillin and streptomycin into cell growth media became common in the 1950s. Penicillin and streptomycin prevent the growth of Gram-positive and Gram-negative bacteria.

Biological fluids and embryo extracts are particularly vulnerable to bacterial contamination. Supplementation with antibiotics reduced this problem. This is an option favored by many laboratories. However, there is a danger that the use of antibiotics may mask a contamination for a short time without eliminating it. This has the effect of delaying a problem rather than removing it. For this reason antibiotics are not used as extensively as in the past. If your aseptic technique is good, then antibiotics should not be required (see Section 5.3 for use of antibiotics).

2.2   How to recognize a contaminated culture

Bacteria and fungi are the main contaminants of mammalian cell cultures. A culture contamination is usually observed by a sudden drop in pH (for some bacterial contaminants) and/or a cloudiness in the medium. If the culture becomes cloudy overnight and changes from red to yellow, it is likely to be contaminated. The color change is associated with a decrease in pH which is indicated by the presence of phenol red in the medium. Under the microscope (at $\times 100$) some granulation may be observed between cells, although it is important to distinguish this from precipitates that may occur from the media, particularly in the presence of serum. At a magnification of $\times 400$ it may be possible to resolve individual bacteria, but unless the contamination is persistent it is not usually necessary to characterize it.

Contamination of cultures with mycoplasma may become a problem. Mycoplasmas derive from a genus of simple prokaryotes with a diameter of $0.2-2$ μm. They have a restricted metabolism and are commonly associated with mammalian cells. They can be elusive because of their potential to pass through filters and they are not visible under low-power microscopy. Furthermore, the normal cocktail of penicillin and streptomycin used in cultures is ineffective because mycoplasmas do not have a cell wall. They are slow growing and consequently may not overgrow the cell culture. However, they may well affect the cellular growth rate, morphology, viability and metabolism.

Mycoplasma infects the cytoplasm of mammalian cells and may cause particularly recognizable effects on metabolism. For example, *Mycoplasma arginini* has a high requirement for arginine and will cause a rapid increase in culture pH. The best way to ensure a mycoplasma-free cell line is to test for mycoplasma contamination at regular intervals – every 3–6 months would be reasonable but this would depend upon usage. The test should be performed in an independent laboratory, so that positive controls could be used and the interpretation of results would be free of bias. Several commercial companies offer a service for mycoplasma testing. One type of test involves the use of fluorescent dyes specific for DNA such as Hoechst 33258 or DAPI (4′,6-diamidino-2-phenylindole). Contaminated cells are identified by microscopic examination for the presence of fluorescent structures in the cytoplasm surrounding a stained cell nucleus (Chen, 1977).

If mycoplasma is detected, the best procedure is to autoclave the contaminated culture and decontaminate the culture laboratory. If the contaminated cells are irreplaceable elimination of the mycoplasma is possible by a cocktail of selected antibiotics, the composition of which depends upon the mycoplasma species. However, such a procedure of cell line decontamination is not always successful.

2.3   What to do if cultures become contaminated?

It is important that contaminated cultures are removed quickly from a culture laboratory before the contamination spreads to noninfected cultures. The cultures should be disinfected and autoclaved as soon as possible and without exposing the sterile area to an infected aerosol.

If stock cells are infected with mycoplasma then they also should be removed from the laboratory and destroyed. Techniques are available to eliminate mycoplasma contamination from cells by selective antibiotic treatment but the procedures are time consuming and only worth consideration if the cell stocks are irreplaceable (Schmidt and Erfle, 1984).

The source of contamination is only worth investigation if the occurrence is frequent. Media contamination may be traced to faulty sterilization or storage in contaminated bottles. With inexperienced workers in cell culture the most probable source of contamination is from poor aseptic technique during culture manipulations.

3.   Culture conditions

Most cells in culture grow best at 37°C and at pH 7.4. If the cells are subjected to a temperature slightly lower than the 37°C optimum then the growth rate will be reduced but the cells should not be damaged. However, higher temperatures of 39–40°C will destroy the cells. So it is very important to be sure that the temperature does not increase in the incubator.

The pH of cultures is maintained by a bicarbonate–CO_2 buffer system which is the main system that operates in blood *in vivo*.

$$CO_2 + H_2O \rightleftharpoons HCO_3^- + H^+$$

The pK_a of this buffering system is 6.3, which is adequate but not ideal for maintaining cultures at pH 7.4, which is the usual optimum for cell growth. The buffer equilibrium in the liquid phase is dependent on the presence of CO_2 in the gas phase. For pH control, an enriched CO_2 atmosphere is provided in the incubator.

A concentration of bicarbonate in the medium (normally 24 mM) maintains an equilibrium with CO_2 at a partial pressure in the gas phase of 40 mmHg (which corresponds to 5% CO_2). In some media formulations the bicarbonate concentration is higher (up to 48 mM). This increases the buffering of the media. However, the CO_2 in the atmosphere has to be set at 10% in order to maintain the pH of the cultures. DMEM cultures are grown in 10% CO_2. EMEM and RPMI cultures are grown in 5% CO_2. The relationship between bicarbonate concentration and gaseous CO_2 is shown in *Table 3.1*.

Even with the bicarbonate–CO_2 buffer system the culture may still undergo pH changes during cell growth. In the early stages of culture a slight increase of pH may occur as a result of bicarbonate decomposition in the medium. However, as the cells grow and energy metabolism becomes well established, the production of lactic acid by cellular metabolism can cause a gradual decline in pH. This drift in culture pH during cell growth should not exceed a pH range of 6.8–7.6. The pH changes can be monitored by the color of phenol red which is normally present in the culture medium. Colors of phenol red:

pH 6.5 = yellow; pH 7.0 = orange; pH 7.4 = red; pH 7.8 = purple

4. Culture medium

Cells are cultured in a chemically complex liquid medium suitable for supporting growth for several generations. There are many standard media formulations that have been developed for the growth of particular cell types (*Table 4.1*).

To determine which media to use for a specific cell line, it is advisable to search the literature to see if previous experiments suggest the use of a particular media formulation. Alternatively, growth trials using three or four different media formulations may be performed. Some media, such as DMEM, have high concentrations of amino acids and vitamins and are suitable for prolonged cell growth. Other media, such as Ham's F-12, contain a wide range of different components which may be required to satisfy the fastidious requirements of some cell lines. Combinations of standard formulations can also be used for cell growth. For example, a 1:1 v/v mixture of DMEM and Ham's F-12 has been found to be effective as a good basal medium for serum-free formulations to support the growth of a number of cell lines.

Media can be supplied commercially as a 1× liquid ready for use or as a concentrate in liquid or powdered form. The concentrates are much cheaper and are advisable if it is intended to use large volumes of one type of medium. The liquid concentrate (normally 10×) is provided sterile and requires dilution with presterilized distilled water. Powdered medium should be dissolved in water and sterilized by filtration through a 0.22 μm filter. Filtration can be mediated by suction with a vacuum pump (*Figure 4.3*) or by liquid pressure from a peristaltic pump (*Figure 4.4*). The systems shown can be bought as presterilized disposable units. The water used for dilution has to be of high purity and should be prepared by reversed osmosis or double distillation. There are some unstable components (e.g. glutamine, bicarbonate) in culture medium and so complete liquid medium

Table 4.1. Commonly used culture media

Media	Comments
BME	Eagle's basal medium; originally designed for mouse L and HeLa cells
EMEM	Eagle's minimum essential medium; used for a wide variety of cell lines
DMEM	Dulbecco's modification of Eagle's medium; has 4× the amino acid and vitamin concentration of BME
GMEM	Glasgow's modification of Eagle's medium; has 2× the amino acid and vitamin concentration of BME
RPMI 1640	Roswell Park Memorial Institute medium; used for lymphocyte and hybridoma cultures
Leibovitz	Used for fibroblast growth in the absence of a CO_2-enriched atmosphere
Ham's F-12	Has a complex composition and used for a variety of cell lines
199	Extremely complex medium (61 components) and can support cell growth without serum

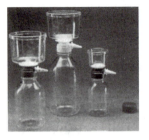

Figure 4.3

Filtration units requiring a vacuum pump.

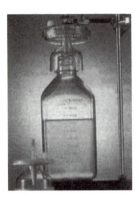

Figure 4.4

Filtration unit through which media is passed from a peristaltic pump.

should not be autoclaved or stored for any length of time. The half-life for glutamine in medium at 4°C is 3 weeks. Liquid medium can be purchased free of glutamine or bicarbonate. In this condition it can be stored at 4°C until required.

4.1   What are the components of a typical culture medium?

- Carbohydrates. Glucose is used in most formulations to provide an energy source as well as a precursor for biosynthesis, such as ribose needed in nucleic acid synthesis. Lactic acid is the major product of glycolysis. In most cultures only a small proportion of glucose is completely oxidized via the tricarboxylic acid (TCA) cycle.

- Alternative carbohydrates may be used, such as fructose, which results in a decreased lactic acid production and a more stable culture pH.

- Amino acids are included at a concentration of 0.1–0.2 mM as a source of precursors for protein synthesis. Glutamine is normally included at higher concentrations (2–4 mM) in order to act as a precursor for the TCA cycle intermediates. However, ammonia is formed from the metabolic breakdown of glutamine and can be inhibitory to growth in some cultures. *Figure 4.5* shows a typical pattern of substrate utilization and by-product formation in a hybridoma culture. The ammonia is produced from glutamine either by thermal degradation in the medium or by cellular metabolism (*Figure 4.6*).

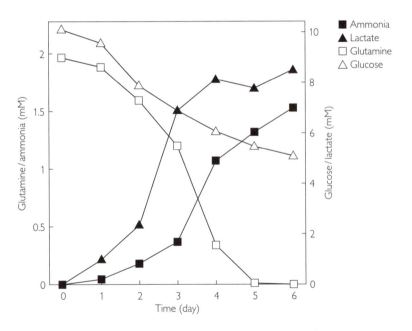

Figure 4.5

Substrate utilization and by-product formation during the growth of a murine hybridoma.

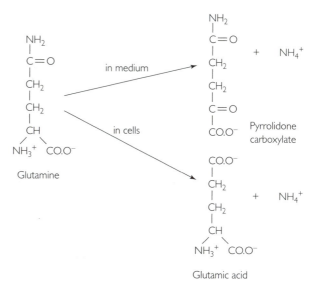

Figure 4.6

Glutamine breakdown in cells and media.

- Salts are included so that the solution is isotonic and has no imbalances with the intracellular content. Osmolarity is a measure of the total number of particles dissolved in a solution.

$$\text{Osmolarity} = \text{molarity} \times \frac{\text{moles of particles or ions}}{\text{moles of solute}}$$

Therefore, a solution at 1 Osmolar (or 1 Osm/l) has 6.023×10^{23} particles in 1 liter of water. Ionization increases the potential number of osmotically active particles. Therefore, 1 mM NaCl = 2 mOsm/l. Osmolality = mOsm/kg of water and is defined by a colligative property such as the ability to reduce the freezing point of water. Thus, a 1 Osm/kg solution reduces the freezing point of water by 0.001858°C. For practical purposes, there is very little difference between osmolarity and osmolality and both terms are used in the cell culture literature.

The osmolarity of standard culture medium is approximately 300 mOsm/l and is optimal for most cell lines. Cells should normally be maintained within 10% of this value. At high osmolarity (>400 mOsm/l), the plating efficiency of cells drops significantly. Lower osmolarity is less damaging although it can result in lower growth rates. Care should be taken in adding supplements to the media or in batch-feeding when the osmolarity may increase significantly.

- Bicarbonate is usually included to act as a buffer system in conjunction with a gaseous atmosphere of 5–10% carbon dioxide provided by the incubator. This allows cultures to be maintained at a pH range of 6.9–7.4. The disadvantage of the bicarbonate–CO_2 buffer system is that cultures may become alkaline very quickly when removed from the incubator. To prevent this or to increase the buffering capacity of the culture, the organic buffer HEPES (pK_a = 7.3 at 37°C) may be added at a concentration of 10–20 mM. HEPES is one of a series of good buffers, that are all organic compounds suitable for buffering at values around their pK. Other examples are MES (pK_a = 6.5), and CHES (pK_a = 9.5). HEPES is the optimal of these for cell culture and it has the advantage that cultures can be grown without an enriched CO_2 atmosphere.

■   Vitamins and hormones are present at relatively low concentrations (μmolar quantities) and are utilized as metabolic co-factors. The content of vitamins and hormones varies enormously from one medium formulation to another. This reflects the variable requirement of cell lines for these components.

■   Phenol red is usually added as a pH indicator of the medium and accounts for the color of culture media. This indicator is useful because it is particularly sensitive to slight pH changes around the growth optimum for cells. At lower pH the phenol red becomes orange (pH 7.0) or yellow (pH 6.5). An overnight change in color of the culture from red to yellow usually indicates bacterial contamination.

5.   Media supplements

5.1   Serum

Serum is normally added to culture media at a concentration of 10% (v/v) to promote cell growth. Serum is the supernatant of clotted blood which contains undefined materials essential for cell proliferation.

Cow (bovine) or horse (equine) serum is most commonly used with fetal calf serum (FCS) being considered particularly effective because of its high content of embryonic growth factors. *Table 4.2* lists some of the characteristics of bovine serum. FCS will promote the growth of a wide range of cell lines, although the availability of this serum can vary. Other suitable bovine sources are 'newborn calf serum' that is processed from an animal under 10 days of age or 'donor calf serum' that is processed from calves under 8 months. Donor horse serum is also widely used in cell culture.

Serum is purchased for laboratory use in 100 ml or 500 ml bottles from a cell culture supplier who will have treated the serum in a particular way. Typically serum is sterilized by filtration through at least one 0.1 μm filter. Each batch is then tested for a variety of microbial and chemical contaminants including bacteria, fungi and specific viruses depending upon the source of the serum.

Special treatment of serum offered by suppliers may include the following.

Table 4.2. Typical characteristics of bovine serum

pH	Osmolarity (mOsm/l)	Protein content (mg/ml)	Albumin content (mg/ml)
6.85–7.05	250–295	60–80	30–50

■ Gamma irradiation involves exposure of the serum to radiation from a ^{60}Co source.

■ Heat inactivation involves incubation at 56°C for 30 minutes.

■ Gamma globulin removal involves ethanol fractionation which reduces the γ-globulin content of the serum. This is important for monoclonal antibody production from hybridoma cultures because γ-globulin derived from serum could interfere with the extraction or assay of the antibody.

■ Dialysis usually involves serum dialysis against 0.15 M NaCl. This reduces the low-molecular-weight components of the serum but maintains its osmolarity. This treatment eliminates the amino acid, carbohydrate or nucleotide content of serum and might be required, for example, in a study of nutrient utilization of cells in culture.

FCS is the most widely used media supplement. However, it is expensive and often in short supply. The serum is generally tested for performance and cytotoxicity. Performance is measured by the ability of the serum to support plating efficiency and cell growth. The specifics of these tests are given by each manufacturer.

5.2   Are there alternatives to serum?

Although serum has been used extensively as a medium supplement to enhance cell growth, there are a number of widely recognized disadvantages connected with its use.

■ It is chemically undefined and variation between batches can result in inconsistent promotion of cell growth.

■ It is expensive. FCS can account for 70–80% of the cost of some formulations. This is an important consideration in large-scale cultures.

■ The proteins in serum can compromise the extraction and purification procedures for cell-secreted proteins.

■ Serum is vulnerable to contamination with infectious agents such as viruses and prions.

For these reasons considerable efforts have been made to develop supplements of hormones and growth factors to replace serum. These serum-free supplements are specific for particular cell types. Commonly used ingredients for these supplements include insulin, transferrin, ethanolamine and selenite. Preprepared serum-free media supplements are commercially available but although these are chemically defined, the manufacturers do not usually reveal the content. Any contaminants are more toxic to cells in low protein medium. So, serum-free formulations must be prepared in water of high purity.

For an extended study on a particular cell line, it is often worth spending some time developing a serum-free formulation based on a modification of a standard published recipe. When developing a serum-free formulation, it is very important to start with an optimal basal medium – rich formulations such as DMEM/Ham's F-12 have been found particularly suitable (see *Table 4.3*).

A gradual process of adaptation of cells from serum to serum-free medium may be necessary depending upon the cell line. To do this, cells are

Table 4.3. A serum-free formulation used for growth of hybridomas

DMEM/Ham's F-12 (1:1 v/v)	
Insulin	5 µg/ml
Transferrin	35 µg/ml
Ethanolamine	20 µM
Sodium selenite	1 nM

From: Murakami, H., et al. (1982) Growth of hybridoma cells in serum-free medium: ethanolamine is an essential component. *Proc Natl. Acad. Sci.* **79**, 1158.
This type of formulation is commonly used for the culture of antibody-secreting hybridomas. The medium supports vigorous cell growth and has the advantage of having a low protein content which is an advantage in antibody extraction.

subcultured in successive media that contain reduced levels of serum. Eventually the medium is replaced by a serum-free formulation.

5.3   Antibiotics

Antibiotics are often included in media for short-term cultures in order to reduce the risk of contamination. The optimal concentration of antibiotics should be determined empirically bearing in mind that they may be cyto-toxic. Antibiotics are often used in combination in culture medium and the following cocktail can be recommended for general use:

- penicillin G (100 U/ml) to inhibit the growth of Gram-positive bacteria;
- streptomycin (50 mg/l) to inhibit the growth of many Gram-negative and Gram-positive bacteria;
- amphotericin B (25 mg/l) as an antifungal agent.

However, the use of antibiotics for routine subculture or in stock cultures should be discouraged because low levels of bacterial or fungal contamination may be masked and may cause problems at a later date. Furthermore, extensive use of antibiotics may cause the selective retention of antibiotic-resistant contaminants which can cause future problems.

6.   Cell metabolism during culture

Figure 4.5 shows the changes in concentration of some of the major components of culture medium during cell growth. Glucose is normally present at an initial concentration of 10–25 mM in most media formulations and this decreases to around half the concentration level within the period of a batch culture. The major role of glucose is to provide the energy metabolism of the cells which occurs primarily anaerobically. The terminal product of glycoly-sis is lactic acid and this is reflected by an accumulation of this compound in the media to parallel the consumption of glucose. The molar ratio of lactate produced/glucose consumed may approach two and this is indicative of anaerobic glycolysis. The production of lactic acid may lower the pH of the culture and this may decrease the cellular growth rate. However, if the culture is appropriately buffered then the accumulated lactate that typically occurs in a batch culture should not cause any growth inhibition.

A secondary but very important function of glucose is to provide a substrate for the pentose phosphate pathway which provides the ribose necessary for nucleic acid synthesis. In fact, it has been shown in some cell cultures that glucose is not essential for cell growth providing there is an alternative source of ribose. Substitution of glucose by either fructose, galactose or maltose decreases the glycolytic rate and production of lactic acid. The metabolism of these alternative carbohydrate sources may proceed exclusively through the pentose phosphate pathway.

Next to the carbohydrate source, glutamine is the most abundant source of reduced carbon in the culture medium. Glutamine is normally included at a concentration of 1–5 mM, which is a significantly higher concentration than any of the other amino acids. Glutamine is an important precursor for the synthesis of purines, pyrimidines, amino sugars and asparagine. However, glutamine also has an important role as substrate for the TCA cycle and this is reflected in a high rate of utilization as shown in *Figure 4.5*. The metabolic pathway for glutamine utilization (called glutaminolysis) follows two steps of nitrogen removal before conversion to 2-oxoglutarate (also known as alpha keto glutarate) which is an intermediate of the TCA cycle. Complete oxidation may occur although it is also likely that other products such as lactic acid or alanine may be by-products of this pathway.

The metabolic deamination of glutamine leads to ammonia which accumulates in the culture up to 2–4 mM and can be inhibitory to cell growth. The problem of ammonia accumulation is made worse by the fact that glutamine may decompose spontaneously to produce ammonia in the culture medium at a rate of 0.1 mM per day at 37°C (*Figure 4.6*). The extent of growth inhibition of ammonia is greater at higher pH and is cell line dependent. Substitution of an alternative carbon source such as glutamate may be possible and will result in a lower production of ammonia. However, cells require adaptation to enable an enhancement of the specific rate of membrane transport, which is normally low for glutamate. The accumulation of ammonia from glutamine can be decreased by a continuous feed of a low concentration of glutamine into the culture or alternatively by the use of glutamine-containing dipeptides that hydrolyze slowly in the culture.

Figure 4.7 shows typical data for the utilization and production of amino acids in cell culture. The mixtures of defined amino acids are normally added to culture media as precursors for protein biosynthesis. However, the figure shows the high rate of glutamine utilization required as an energy source and the significant release of alanine into the medium by cells. The accumulation of alanine is a reflection of a mechanism of sequestration (or detoxification) of ammonia in the cell by amination of pyruvate, produced by glycolysis or by glutaminolysis. The accumulated alanine is not growth inhibitory and may in fact be utilized toward the end of the culture if the supply of other carbon sources decreases. Of the other amino acids, serine, aspartic acid and those with a branched chain are particularly well utilized. The sulfur-containing amino acids methionine and cysteine are essential and rapidly consumed.

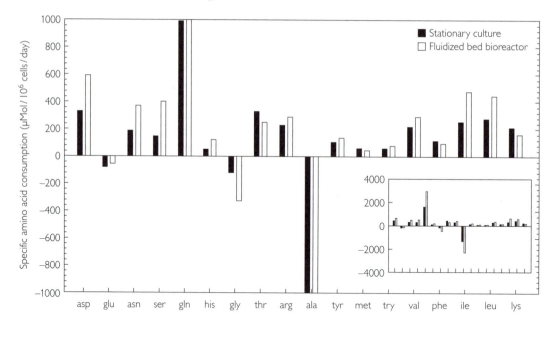

Figure 4.7

Specific amino acid consumption in two cultures.

References

Chen, T.R. (1977) In situ demonstration of mycoplasma contamination in cell cultures by fluorescent Hoechst 33258 stain. *Exp. Cell Res.* **104**: 255–262.

Cotter, T.G. and Al-Rubeai, M. (1995) Cell death (apoptosis) in cell culture systems. *Trends Biotechnol.* **13**: 150–155.

Murakami, H., Masui, H., Sato, G.H., Sueoka, N., Chow, T.P. and Kano-Sueoka, T. (1982) Growth of hybridoma cells in serum-free medium: ethanolamine is an essential component. *Proc. Natl Acad. Sci.* **79**: 1158–1162.

Rous, P. and Jones, F.S. (1916) A method for obtaining suspension of living cells from the fixed tissues for the plating out of individual cells. *J. Exp. Med.* **23**: 546.

Schmidt, J. and Erfle, V. (1984) Elimination of mycoplasma from cell cultures and establishment of mycoplasma-free cell lines. *Exp. Cell Res.* **152**: 565–570.

Further reading

Detailed protocols for handling laboratory-scale cell cultures are included in the following general texts.

Adams, L.P. (1980) *Cell Culture for Biochemists: Laboratory Techniques in Biochemistry and Molecular Biology*. Elsevier, Barking.

Butler, M. (ed.) (1991) *Mammalian Cell Biotechnology: A Practical Approach*. Oxford University Press, Oxford.

Fogh, J. (ed.) (1973) *Contamination in Tissue Culture*. Academic Press, New York.

Freshney, R.I. (1992) *Animal Cell Culture: a Practical Approach*, 2nd Edn. IRL Press, Oxford.

Freshney, R.I. (1994) *Culture of Animal Cells: A Manual of Basic Technique*. A.R. Liss, New York.

Jakoby, W.B. and Pastan, I.H. (eds) (1979) *'Cell Culture' Methods in Enzymology LVIII*. Academic Press, New York.

McGarrity, G.J., Murphy, D.G. and Nichols, W.W. (eds) (1978) *Mycoplasma Infection in Cell Cultures*. Plenum Press, New York.

Morgan, S.J. and Darling, D.C. (1993) *Animal Cell Culture*. BIOS Scientific, Oxford.

Paul, J. (1975) *Cell and Tissue Culture*. Livingstone, Edinburgh.

Spier, R.E. and Griffiths, B. (eds) (1986–1994) *Animal Cell Biotechnology*, Vols 1–6. Academic Press, London.

Protocol 4.1

Harvesting anchorage-dependent cells with trypsin

Reagent

Trypsin reagent: 4 ml trypsin (0.25%) + 16 ml versene in 0.2 g/l PBS

Method

1. Remove growth medium from culture flask by decanting or with a suction pump.

2. Wash cells in flask with PBS.

3. Add trypsin/versene reagent to completely cover the cell layer.

4. Incubate at 37°C for up to 15 min. Examine the cell layer at frequent intervals. Tap the flask gently to aid the dispersion of cells.

5. When the cell sheet is sufficiently dispersed, add growth medium (with serum) or trypsin inhibitor. Use approximately ×5 volume of trypsin solution left on the cells.

6. Transfer cell suspension into fresh medium. Dispense into new flasks – the subcultures.

Protocol 4.2

Adaptation of cells to a serum-free medium

Introduction

Some cell lines can be subcultured directly from a serum-based to a serum-free medium without loss of growth performance. However, in other cases cells may be adapted slowly into the new serum-free medium. The process of adaptation may involve changes in cellular metabolism or the induction of specific cellular growth factors. The following protocol is suitable in allowing such changes as cells are weaned to a new medium.

Method

1. Anchorage-dependent cells such as MDCK grow well in a medium such as DMEM supplemented with 5% calf serum. This can be used as a starting culture for adaptation to the serum-free medium (SFM).

2. Inoculate cells grown in the serum-based medium (SBM) into a medium containing 5:1 v/v SBM: SFM at a density $>2 \times 10^5$ cells/ml.

3. Subculture after 48 h growth for two passages.

4. Increase the content of serum-free medium by changing the SBM/SFM ratio to 4:1, 3:1, 2:1, 1:1, 1:2, 1:3, 1:5 and 1:10 before growing in 100% SFM. At each stage of medium dilution subculture ($\times$2) as in step 3.

5. It may be necessary to repeat some of the steps of adaptation if cell growth is poor. This may occur at low levels of serum.

Protocol 4.3

The trypsinization of cells in serum-free medium

Introduction

During the subculture of anchorage-dependent cells, the proteolytic activity of trypsin is used to detach cells from the surface of a culture flask. The exposure of MDCK cells to trypsin should be as short as possible (typically 20 min) to minimize the potential of proteolytic damage of the cells. In serum-supplemented cultures the addition of fresh medium is sufficient to neutralize the effect of the trypsin because of the high protein content. However, in low-protein serum-free media the trypsin must be neutralized by use of a specific inhibitor prior to subculture.

The method described below allows subculture with trypsin but without the requirement for serum.

Materials

Trypsin inhibitor: 0.25% w/v soybean trypsin inhibitor (Gibco-BRL 17075–029) in Dulbecco's phosphate buffered saline (filter sterilized).

Method

1.   Remove media from a 75 cm² T-flask and add 8 ml prewarmed PBS-EDTA.

2.   Let the flask stand for 30 seconds then remove the PBS-EDTA.

3.   Add 1.5 ml prewarmed trypsin (0.25%). Incubate for 10–20 min at 37°C. Gently tilt the flask every few minutes to distribute the trypsin evenly.

4.   The translucent monolayer should become more opaque. When this occurs tap the flask firmly 10 times against the palm of the hand to dislodge the monolayer of cells. If the cells do not dislodge continue to incubate them at 37°C.

5.   Add 2.0 ml trypsin inhibitor 0.25%, swirl the flask and let stand for 1 minute.

6.   Add 8 ml PBS-EDTA and break up the aggregates by pipetting up and down 10–20 times. Centrifuge at 300 g for 5 min.

7.   Aspirate the supernatant and re-suspend the cells in an appropriate amount of prewarmed media – usually at 10^5 cells/ml to initiate a new culture.

Note

The quantity or concentration of trypsin addition may be varied depending on the cells and how firmly they are attached to the growth surface. It is recommended to use the same volume and concentration of trypsin inhibitor at stage 5 as trypsin used at stage 3.

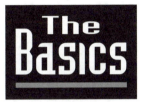

Chapter 5

Cell line and culture monitoring

1. Cell counting and monitoring

Growth in cultures is normally determined by counting cells at regular intervals. In routine cultures this would be performed once a day, which corresponds to the approximate doubling time of mammalian cells during the exponential growth phase. This would establish an overall growth profile of a culture. More frequent counts would be required to follow more subtle changes that may, for example, be associated with the cell growth cycle.

In addition to this, it is worthwhile inspecting cultures under a microscope to determine if there are any significant changes to the appearance of the cells. The two microscope types used for monitoring cells are described in Chapter 3.

Growth in cultures is normally determined by counting cells at regular intervals – at least once a day. The two direct methods commonly used are manual counting through a microscope or electronic counting by a particle counter. Both methods depend upon obtaining a sample of an even distribution of cells in suspension. Therefore it is extremely important to ensure that the culture is well mixed by stirring or shaking before taking a sample.

1.1 Hemocytometer

This is a thick glass plate which fits onto the adjustable stage of a microscope. There are several designs available (Burker, Fuchs-Rosenthal and Neubauer). The most common type used is the improved Neubauer. Through the microscope you can see a grooved calibrated grid on the hemocytometer surface (*Figure 5.1*). This consists of nine large squares with 1 mm sides. The central square is subdivided into 25 squares each of which is further subdivided into 16 squares of 0.05×0.05 mm. A cell suspension is put onto the grid by touching the end of a capillary tube containing the cell suspension at the edge of a cover slip placed on the upper surface of the hemocytometer. The position of the cover slip forms a chamber, the sides of which are the calibrated edges of the slide raised exactly 0.1 mm above the ruled surface. The volume contained in each of the nine large squares is $1 \times 1 \times 0.1 = 0.1$ mm^3 ($= 0.1$ µl). The cells are then counted in a standard volume (usually 5×0.1 µl) as defined by the area of the grid. In this case:

$$\text{cells per ml} = \frac{\text{Total count} \times 10^4}{5}$$

A standard microscope at low magnification of $\times 40$ to $\times 100$ is required for viewing the cells. A hand-held tally counter helps in counting. This is shown in *Figure 5.2* with a standard hemocytometer (*Protocol 5.1*).

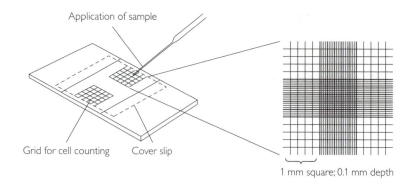

Application of sample

Grid for cell counting   Cover slip

1 mm square; 0.1 mm depth

Figure 5.1

Hemocytometer.

Trypan blue is often added to the cell suspension before counting. The dye penetrates the membrane of nonviable cells which are stained blue and which can therefore be distinguished from viable cells (Patterson, 1979). Viability gives an indication of the ability of a cell to divide (see Section 3). The viability is usually expressed as a percentage of viable cells in a population.

% viability = (number of viable cells/total number of cells) × 100

This is the most commonly used assay for cell viability.

A modification of this method involves counting nuclei (*Protocol 5.2*). Incubation of cell samples in a mixture of citric acid and crystal violet causes cells to lyse and the released nuclei to stain purple (Sanford *et al.*, 1951). Nuclei counting is well suited to the determination of anchorage-dependent cells, for example when attached to microcarriers. However, care must be taken in interpreting nuclei counts as cells can become binucleated, particularly when growth is arrested. As a result the nuclei concentration may be higher than the cell concentration (Berry *et al.*, 1996).

The hemocytometer counting method is simple and effective but can be laborious if many samples are being analyzed. The expected error in cell concentration is around 10%. This can arise from variability in sampling, dilution, mixing, filling the chamber or counting.

1.2   Coulter counter

An electronic cell counter (or Coulter counter) is suitable for rapid counting of multiple samples of cells in suspension (*Figure 5.3*). The principle of the counter is that a predetermined volume (usually 0.5 ml) of a cell suspension diluted in buffered saline is forced through a small hole (diameter 70 μm) in a tube by suction. The cells (or any particles) cause a measurable change in electrical resistance as they pass between two electrodes, one inside and one outside the glass tube. This produces a series of pulses recorded as a signal on an oscilloscope. Several thousand particles per second may be counted and sized with accuracy.

In the simplest instrument (e.g. Coulter model D Industrial) a lower size threshold of counting may be set electronically (*Figure 5.4*). Thus, particles smaller than cells (dust or cell fragments) can be eliminated from the count.

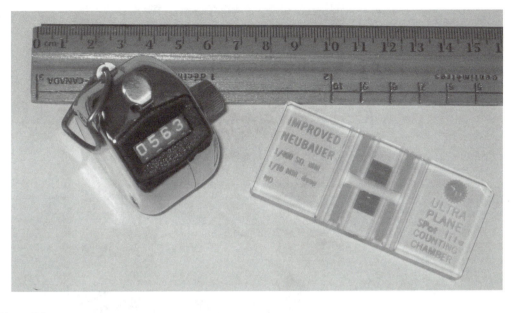

Figure 5.2

Improved Neubauer hemocytometer with tally counter. Courtesy of Beckman Coulter Ltd.

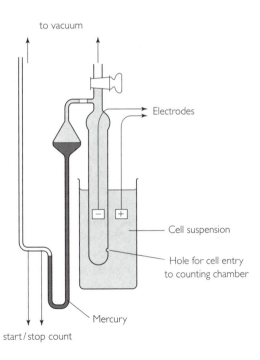

Figure 5.3

The principle of the Coulter counter.

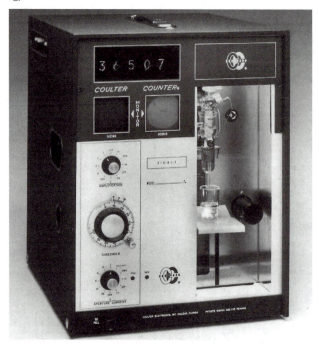

Figure 5.4

Coulter counter.

The largest particle size is determined by the size of the orifice in the tube, which is normally 75 or 100 μm. For routine counting the Coulter Industrial D is more than adequate. In more complex instruments (e.g. Coulter model ZB) a lower and upper size threshold ('gates') can be set electronically. This allows the size distribution of a cell population to be determined. Particles smaller than cells can be eliminated from the count by setting a lower threshold of detection. The largest particle size is determined by the size of the hole in the tube. The size distribution of a cell population can be determined by changing the threshold setting of the Coulter counter (*Protocol 5.3*). This requires a size calibration with a standard suspension of particles such as latex beads or pollen grains.

The major advantage of this method is the speed of analysis and therefore the suitability for counting a large number of samples. It is also reasonably accurate within an expected counting error of less than 5%. However, the method is based upon the number of particles contained in suspension and, consequently, the proportion of viable cells in the sample cannot be determined. Also, it must be ensured that cell aggregates are not present in the sample; otherwise the cell count will be underestimated. Cell suspensions above 10^4 per ml should be diluted otherwise two or more cells passing through the counting zone at the same time will cause coincidence errors. A standard protocol is to dilute a cell suspension ($\times20$–40) in a saline solution (Isoton).

2.   Indirect methods of cell determination

Indirect methods of estimating cell growth rely on the measurement of an intracellular cell component such as DNA or protein or alternatively an extracellular change such as nutrient depletion or an enzyme activity released by the cells. Indirect methods of growth estimation depend upon a correlation between the measured parameter and cell concentration. However, it is important to realize that these relationships are rarely linear over the course of a culture. It is well documented that the total protein content and specific enzyme activity levels measured on a per cell basis vary substantially over the course of a culture due to changes in the growth rate and composition of the culture medium. For example, the protein and enzyme content per cell will be high during exponential growth but lower in the lag or stationary phases.

In some situations, as may occur for example in immobilized cell bioreactor systems, an indirect measurement of cell growth may be the only option available. This can be used to monitor the progress of a culture. However, care must be taken if such data are used in comparative analysis between cultures, as differences may be a reflection of changes in metabolic or functional activity rather than of cell concentration.

There are a number of colorimetric methods based on the measurement of cell components. These are relatively simple methods and suitable for multiple samples.

2.1   Protein determination

Total cell protein can be used as a measure of biomass (total cellular material) but the protein content per cell can vary during cell culture and this can be a reflection of changing cell size (*Protocol 5.4*). The protein content of a mammalian cell is typically 100–500 pg/cell. These measurements are also useful in the expression of specific enzyme activities which are commonly expressed as the maximum measured reaction velocity of an enzyme per total cell protein.

The most sensitive colorimetric assays are the Lowry and Bradford methods. Of these the Bradford assay is favored because of speed, sensitivity and negligible interference from other cell components (Bradford, 1976). By this method, lysed cells are solubilized in NaOH and added to the reagent, Coomassie blue. A blue color which develops within 10 min can be measured by a colorimeter or spectrophotometer and compared with standard proteins.

2.2   DNA determination

The DNA content of diploid cells is usually constant, although variations can occur as a result of the distribution of cells through the cell cycle (*Protocol 5.5*). Cells in the G1 phase have the normal diploid content of DNA, which is typically 6 pg per cell (see Section 5 for analysis of phases of cell cycle).

DNA measurement is probably the best method to use as an indicator of the number of cells in a solid tissue (Labarca and Paigen, 1980). A commonly used method involves treatment of the solubilized cells with diphenylamine reagent which forms a blue coloration with DNA. Fluorescence detection (Kurtz and Wells, 1979) can also be used with Hoechst 33258 or DAPI (Brunk et al., 1979), which bind to DNA (see mycoplasma detection; Section 2.2, Chapter 4).

2.3   Glucose determination

If cells are immobilized within a bioreactor, then it is often difficult to obtain a cell sample. Examples of such bioreactors include a packed-bed or hollow fiber system (see Chapter 9).

Cell growth can be monitored by changes in the concentration of key components of the culture medium. The rate of change in the glucose content of the medium may be suitable for such an assay as an indirect measure of cell concentration (*Protocol 5.6*). Alternatives include measurement of lactic acid production or oxygen consumption.

Correlations have been shown between cell concentration and consumption or production of these components. This relationship may be constant for a particular cell line under a given set of conditions. However, if the cell line or any of the culture conditions are altered the relationship between substrate consumption or product formation and cell number will change.

3.   Viability measurements

Viability is a measure of the metabolic state of a cell population, which is indicative of the potential of the cells for growth. This is a measure of the proportion of live, metabolically active cells in a culture, as indicated by the ability of cells to divide or to perform normal metabolism. The viability may be determined from simple assays such as dye exclusion where cells are designated as either viable or nonviable (see Section 1.1). From the dye exclusion method the loss of viability is recognized by membrane damage resulting in the penetration of the dye, trypan blue. Other dyes that can be used include erythrosin B, nigrosin and fluorescein diacetate.

3.1   Tetrazolium assay

The tetrazolium assay is a measure of cellular oxidative metabolism (*Protocol 5.7*). A colorimetric assay for viable cells has been developed (Mosmann, 1983) using the tetrazolium dye, MTT [3-(4,5-dimethylthiazol-2-yl)-2,5-diphenyltetrazolium bromide]. The dye is cleaved to a colored product by the activity of dehydrogenase enzymes and this indicates high levels of mitochondrial activity in cells. The color development (yellow to blue) is proportional to the number of metabolically active cells. However, there is considerable variation in results between cell lines with some cells producing a very low response. Cells with a significant level of oxidative metabolism such as CHO produce a good response in the MTT assay.

The method is particularly convenient for the rapid assay of replicate cell cultures in multi-well plates.

3.2   Lactate dehydrogenase determination

Loss of cell viability may be followed by an increase in enzyme activity in the culture medium caused by a damaged cell membrane which allows large molecules to enter or leave the intracellular pool (*Protocol 5.8*). The activity of lactate dehydrogenase (LDH) is the most commonly measured enzyme in this technique (Wagner *et al.*, 1992). This activity increases as the enzyme escapes through the damaged membrane of nonviable cells. The enzyme activity can be measured easily by a simple spectrophotometric assay involving the oxidation of NADH in the presence of pyruvate. The reaction is monitored by a decrease in UV absorbance at 340 nm.

$$\text{pyruvate} + \text{NADH} + \text{H}^+ \overset{\text{LDH}}{\longleftrightarrow} \text{lactate} + \text{NAD}^+$$

NADH absorbs at $\lambda = 340$ nm.

The specific enzyme activity is defined as the maximum measured reaction velocity of an enzyme per total cell protein. For LDH this equals $\sim 1\text{--}3 \times 10^3$ nmol lactate/min per mg cell protein.

The method is well suited for the determination of multiple samples, particularly if a multi-well plate reader is available. This instrument enables the light absorbance of all wells to be measured within seconds (*Figure 3.9*). However, care must be taken when interpreting the results by this method because the LDH content per cell can change considerably during the course of batch culture. The loss of cell viability can be expressed as the activity of LDH in the medium as a proportion of total LDH in the culture.

3.3   Adenylate energy charge

The energy charge is an index based on the measurement of the intracellular levels of the nucleotides, AMP, ADP, and ATP (*Protocol 5.9*).

$$\text{the energy charge} = \frac{\text{ATP} + 0.5.\text{ADP}}{\text{ATP} + \text{ADP} + \text{AMP}}$$

This is based on the interconversion of the three adenylate nucleotides in the cell:

$$\text{AMP} \leftrightarrow \text{ADP} \leftrightarrow \text{ATP}$$

This index varies between the theoretical limits of 0 and 1. For normal cells, values of 0.7–0.9 would be expected, but a gradual decrease in the value gives an early indication of loss of viability by a cell population. These nucleotide concentrations can be measured by high performance liquid chromatography (HPLC) or by luminescence using the luciferin–luciferase enzyme system (Holm-Hansen and Karl, 1978). Such measurements are not as easy to perform as the routine counting procedures discussed earlier (Section 1) but can be a means of monitoring the decline in the energy metabolism of a cell culture during the loss of viability.

3.4   Rate of protein or nucleic acid synthesis

The metabolic activity of cells can be measured by their rate of protein or DNA synthesis (*Protocol 5.10*). This is based on the incubation of intact cells in standard culture medium to which is added a radioactively labeled amino acid or a nucleotide. Any radioactive amino acid is suitable but those most commonly used are ^{3}H-leucine or ^{35}S-methionine (Dickson, 1991). Nucleic acid synthesis is measured by the utilization of tritiated thymidine (^{3}H-TdR). This is also the basis for the determination of the cell cycle (Section 5.1).

3.5   Colony-forming assay

The most precise of all methods of viability measurement is the colony-forming assay. Here the ability of cells to grow is measured directly (Cook and Mitchell, 1989). A known number of cells at low density is allowed to attach and grow on the surface of a Petri dish. If the cell density is kept low, each viable cell will divide and give rise to a colony or cluster of cells. From this, the 'plating efficiency' is determined as the number of colonies scored per 100 cells plated × 100.

Although the colony-forming assay is time-consuming, it has been used widely in cytotoxicity studies. *Figure 5.5* shows how the effect of treating cells with a potentially toxic compound is determined by a change in the plating efficiency. The colonies of treated cells are compared with controls. The effect of the treatment is assessed by the relative surviving fraction which equals the colonies on treated Petri dish/colonies on untreated Petri dish.

A less precise method of determining the viability by the cellular repro- ductive potential is from the lag phase of a growth curve. *Figure 5.6* shows that, by extrapolation from the linear portion of the growth curve to time zero, the derived cell number can be compared with the original count. This method can be easily adapted to determine how a particular treatment affects cell viability.

4.   Cell line identification

4.1   The need for cell line monitoring

Because different cell lines may be handled in the same laboratory, there is a danger of cross-contamination. This problem became apparent in the 1960s when it was discovered that a variety of widely used cell lines that had been exchanged between laboratories were contaminated with HeLa cells. HeLa are fast-growing cells that are capable of outgrowing most other cell lines. This contamination was so widespread that many cell lines that were originally isolated in the 1960s have been shown to have genetic markers derived from HeLa cells, indicating that DNA exchange occurred at some time (Nelson-Rees *et al.*, 1981).

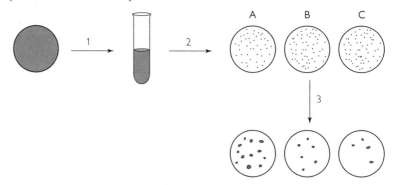

1: Remove the cells from the attachment surface and suspend in media.
2: Add cell suspension to Petri dishes, each may be treated differently. A is the untreated control. B and C are treated with an agent to be tested. Incubate to allow colonies to form.
3: Fix the colonies with methanol/acetic acid and stain with crystal violet.
   The relative surviving fraction is determined from the number of independent colonies in each dish compared to the control. Relative surviving fraction in B=6/12=0.5; in C=4/12=0.33 (from Cook and Mitchell, 1989).

Figure 5.5

Colony-forming assay. (Modified from Cook and Mitchell, 1989.)

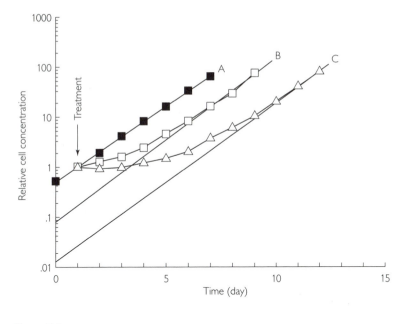

Figure 5.6

Survival assay by extrapolation of a growth curve.

Cell lines that are grown continuously in culture are vulnerable to genetic change. This can arise through intrinsic alteration of the genome of the cultured cells by mutation or by selective pressures. Therefore, cells grown for several passages in culture may be quite different from those originally derived from primary tissue. Because of these reasons, it is important to monitor the genetic characteristics of a continuously growing cell line at regular intervals.

4.2   What tests can be used to identify a cell line?

The following can be used to characterize and assign a unique set of recognition markers for a cell line:

- karyotype;
- isozyme patterns;
- antibody labeling;
- DNA fingerprinting.

Karyotyping

This is used to establish the distribution of chromosomes (karyotype) and may indicate the species of origin of the cells. The chromosome composition can also indicate whether the cells are transformed or whether any chromosome damage has occurred.

Individual chromosomes can be seen under a microscope during mitosis. Chromosome identification can be aided by a banding technique. This involves the use of a dye which generates a reproducible pattern of stained bands on each chromosome. The molecular basis for the development of these bands is not clearly understood but probably relates to areas of highly condensed chromosomal material. One commonly used dye is

Giemsa (Wang and Fedoroff, 1972). In this technique nucleoprotein is partially digested by trypsin, and the Giemsa dye produces a characteristic pattern of G bands (*Protocol 5.11*). *Figure 5.7* shows a typical banding pattern for human chromosomes as viewed under a light microscope. *Figure 5.8* shows the detailed pattern that can be deciphered for the human X-chromosome.

A transformed cell population may be heteroploid, that is, have a chromosome count that varies between individual cells. In order to characterize such a cell line, chromosomes are counted for 100–200 individual cells, and a modal chromosome number is calculated.

Isozymes

The analysis of isozyme patterns of selected enzymes has been used extensively as a technique to identify the species of origin of cell lines with a high degree of certainty (Halton *et al.*, 1983). Isozymes (or isoenzymes) are structurally different forms of the same enzyme. They catalyze the same reaction but have different protein structures.

The technique involves gel electrophoresis of cell homogenates under non-denaturing conditions. Specific activity stains are used to develop a banding pattern of isozymes (zymogram), which is characteristic of a particular cell line. Such zymograms are usually photographed to provide a permanent record of each cell line.

Of the various enzymes that can be separated into isozymes by this technique, glucose 6-phosphate dehydrogenase, lactate dehydrogenase, and nucleoside phosphorylase have been particularly well characterized. By

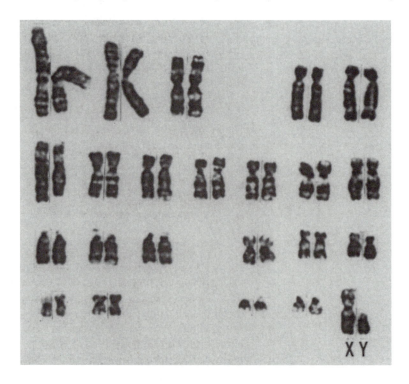

Figure 5.7

Human male karyotype with G-banded chromosomes.

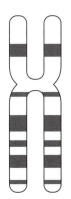

Figure 5.8

*G-bands of a human
X chromosome.*

using several enzymes the distinguishing features of a cell line are established. These features can often distinguish cell lines even if derived from the same species. This is a more rapid technique compared to karyotyping and requires smaller cell samples. *Figure 5.9* shows typical zymogram patterns for selected cell lines.

Labeled antibodies

A cell line can be identified by use of a fluorescent-labeled antibody specific for a membrane antigen. The antibody, prepared by methods described in Chapter 8, is conjugated to a suitable fluorescent compound, such as fluorescein. The conjugate will bind specifically to the outer membrane of the chosen cells which can be identified by fluorescence microscopy or by a fluorescence-activated cell sorter (*Figure 5.13*).

DNA fingerprinting

This technique is well known in forensic science but is gradually being adopted as a standard reference technique for cell line identity in culture collections (Stacey, 1991). A unique DNA 'fingerprint' can be developed for a particular cell line.

The DNA fingerprint results from the fragmentation pattern produced by digestion of cellular DNA with restriction endonucleases. The resulting restriction fragment digest is separated by electrophoresis. Radioactive probes are then used to hybridize to specific restriction fragments which can be highlighted by autoradiography. This results in a characteristic 'bar-code' pattern.

The most useful probes for this purpose are those that hybridize to 'minisatellite' DNA (Jeffreys *et al.*, 1985). These are repetitive nucleotide sequences of varying length found throughout the genomic DNA. Certain restriction enzymes (for example, Hinf1) are used because they are known to cut DNA within the minisatellite regions. The length and distribution of the resulting minisatellite DNA fragments are unique to individuals and hence can be used for identification, including cell line identification.

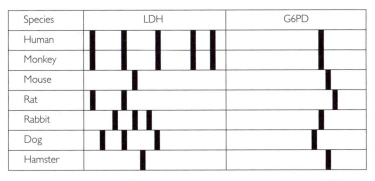

Distinct banding patterns are shown for the enzymes lactate dehydrogenase (LDH) and glucose 6-phosphate dehydrogenase (G6PD) derived from cell lines of different species

Figure 5.9

Zymograms.

5.   Analysis of the cell cycle

During growth, cells go through a series of stages characterized by two major events – DNA synthesis and cell division by mitosis. Any cell population will consist of cells distributed through four phases of the cell cycle – G1 (gap), S (synthesis), G2 (gap) and M (mitosis). The S phase is a period of DNA synthesis, M is a stage of cell division by mitosis, G1 is an uncharacterized phase after mitosis and G2 is an uncharacterized phase after S. The cells at each stage differ in their DNA content – G1 cells have the normal diploid content of DNA. M and G2 cells have ×2 the diploid DNA content and the S cells have a DNA content changing from ×1 to ×2. The length of each phase for a typical population of mammalian cells during growth is given in *Figure 5.10*.

During culture the proportion of cells at each phase of the cycle changes. In the stationary and decline culture phases there is an increased proportion of cells at G1 of the cell cycle. During growth there is a high proportion of cells in the S phase and a low proportion in the G1 phase. The metabolic activity of cells can often be related to cell cycle phase changes. For example, enhanced antibody synthesis has been shown by some lymphocyte hybridomas in the G1 phase.

The following two methods are available to analyze the distribution of a cell population between the phases of the cell cycle.

5.1   Tritiated thymidine pulse method

This method can be used to determine the proportion of cells involved in DNA replication and allows an estimate of the length of the S phase. Cells are incubated in a medium containing ^{3}H-thymidine for a short period of time (~30 min). During this time only cells in the S phase will incorporate radioactivity into the DNA. This is followed by a period (~ 1 h) of incubation in nonradioactive medium. The cells are then fixed on a microscope slide and prepared for autoradiography. This allows the determination of the fraction of cells which have incorporated ^{3}H-thymidine. This fraction multiplied by the total generation time gives the length of the S phase.

5.2   Flow cytometer

This is a sophisticated and expensive piece of equipment which would be found in a specialized laboratory (*Figure 5.11*). The cytometer is capable of analyzing cells treated with a fluorescent stain – for cell cycle analysis the

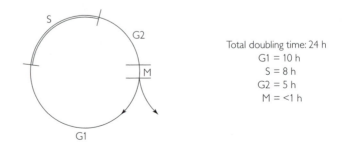

Total doubling time: 24 h
G1 = 10 h
S = 8 h
G2 = 5 h
M = <1 h

Figure 5.10

Cell cycle for a typical population of mammalian cells during exponential growth.

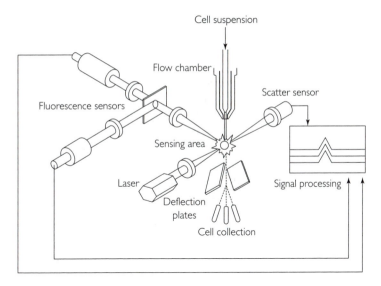

Figure 5.11

Flow cytometer and cell sorter.

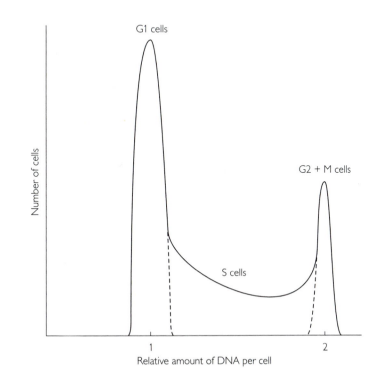

Figure 5.12

Distribution over the four phases of the cell cycle.

stain is specific for DNA. The stained cells are then forced through a fine nozzle at a rate of several thousand cells per second. This stream of cells is exposed to a laser beam and the resulting fluorescence emission is detected by a photomultiplier. Since the fluorescence intensity is directly proportional to the DNA content of each cell, the data output gives a distribution analysis of the cell population by DNA content. This information can be related to the distribution of cells through the cell cycle. *Figure 5.12* shows a typical pattern of results obtained by this method. The G2 + M peak is recognized at ×2 the relative DNA content of the G1 peak, whilst the S phase cells are indicated by the band between the peaks. The integrated areas under the peaks, as defined by the extrapolated dotted lines in *Figure 5.12*, are representative of the proportion of cells in each phase.

A further application of this type of instrument is in fluorescent-activated cell sorting as illustrated in *Figure 5.13*. Cells detected with a fluorescent label may be differentially charged and that allows them to be deflected to a collecting tube following passage through two electrodes.

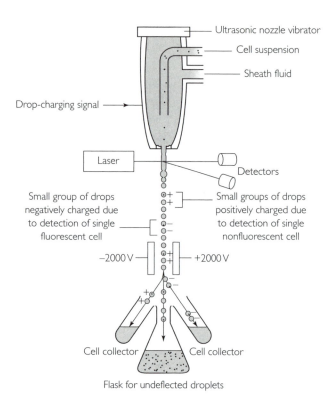

Figure 5.13

Fluorescence-activated cell sorter.

References

Bergmeyer, H.U. and Bernt, E. (1974) Determination with glucose oxidase and peroxidase In: Bergmeyer, H.U. (ed.) *Methods of Enzymatic Analysis* 2nd edn., Volume 3, pp. 1205–1212. VCH, Weinheim.

Berry, J.M., Huebner, E. and Butler, M. (1996). The crystal violet nuclei staining technique leads to anomalous results in monitoring mammalian cell cultures. *Cytotechnology* 21: 73–80.

Bradford, M. (1976) A rapid and sensitive method for the quantitation of microgram quantities of protein using the principle of protein-dye binding. *Anal. Biochem.* 72: 248–254.

Brunk, C.F., Jones, K.C. and James, T.W. (1979) Assay for nanogram quantities of DNA in cellular homogenates. *Anal. Biochem.* 92: 497–500.

Cook, J.A. and Mitchell, J.B. (1989) Viability measurements in mammalian cell systems. *Anal. Biochem.* 179: 1–7.

Dickson, A.J. (1991) Protein expression and processing. In: Butler, M. (ed.) *Mammalian Cell Biotechnology: A Practical Approach*, pp.85–108. Oxford University Press, Oxford.

Halton, D.M., Peterson, W.D.Jr. and Hukku, B. (1983) Cell culture quality control by rapid isoenzymatic characteristics. *In Vitro* 19: 16–24.

Holm-Hansen, O. and Karl, D.M. (1978) Biomass and adenylate energy charge determination in microbial cell extracts and environmental samples. *Methods Enzymol.* 57: 73–85.

Jeffreys, A.J., Wilson, V. and Thein, S.L. (1985) Individual 'fingerprints' of human DNA. *Nature* 316: 76–79.

Kunst, A., Draeger, B. and Ziegenhorn, J. (1984) UV-methods with hexokinase and glucose 6-phosphate dehydrogenase. In: Bergmeyer, H.U. (ed.) *Methods of Enzymatic Analysis*, 3rd edn., Volume 8, pp. 163–172. VCH, Weinheim.

Kurtz, J.W. and Wells, W.W. (1979) Automated fluorometric analysis of DNA, protein and enzyme activities: Application of methods in cell culture. *Anal. Biochem.* 94: 166–175.

Labarca, C. and Paigen, K. (1980) A simple, rapid and sensitive DNA assay procedure. *Anal. Biochem.* 102: 344–352.

Lundin, A., Hasenson, M., Persson, J. and Pousette, A. (1986) Estimation of biomass in growing cell lines by adenosine triphosphate assay. *Methods Enzymol.* 133: 27–42.

Mosmann, T. (1983) Rapid colorimetric assay for cellular growth and survival: application to proliferation and cytotoxicity assays. *J. Immunol. Methods* 65: 55–63.

Nelson-Rees, W.A., Daniels, W. and Flandermeyer, R. (1981) Cross-contamination of cells in culture. *Science* 212: 446–452.

Patterson, M.K. (1979) Measurement of growth and viability of cells in culture. *Methods Enzymol.* 58: 141–152.

Sanford, K.K., Earle, W.R., Evans, V.J., Waltz, H.K. and Shannon, J.E. (1951) The measurement of proliferation in tissue cultures by enumeration of cell nuclei. *J. Natl Cancer Inst.* 11: 773–795.

Stacey, G. (1991) DNA fingerprinting and the characterisation of cell lines. *Cytotechnology* 6: 91–92.

Wagner, A., Marc, A. and Engasser, J.M. (1992) The use of lactate dehydrogenase (LDH) release kinetics for the evaluation of death and growth of mammalian cells in perfusion reactors. *Biotech. Bioeng.* 39: 320–326.

Wang, H.C. and Fedoroff, S. (1972) Banding in human chromosomes treated with trypsin. *Nat. New Biol.* 235: 52–53.

Further reading

Al-Rubeai, M. and Emery, A.N. (1993) Flow Cytometry in Animal Cell Culture. *Biotechnology* 11: 572–579.

Al-Rubeai, M. and Emery, A.N. (eds) (1995) *Flow Cytometry Applications in Cell Culture*. Marcel Dekker, New York.

Baserga, R. (1981) *The Biology of Cell Reproduction*. Harvard University Press, Cambridge, MA.

Doyle, A., Morris, C. and Mowles, J.M. (1990) Quality control. In: Doyle, A., Hay, R. and Kirsop, B.E. *et al.* (eds) *Living Resources for Biotechnology: Animal Cells*, pp. 81–100. Cambridge University Press, Cambridge.

John, P.C.L. (ed.) (1981) *The Cell Cycle*. Cambridge University Press, Cambridge.

King, K.L. and Cidlowski, J.A. (1998) Cell cycle regulation and apoptosis. *Ann. Rev. Physiol.* **60:** 601–617.

Mazia, D. (1974) The cell cycle. *Sci. Am.* **230:** 54–64.

Melamad, M.R., Mullaney, P.F. and Mendelsohn, M.L. (1979) *Flow Cytometry and Sorting*. John Wiley, New York.

Yunis, J. (1974) *Human Chromosome Methodology*. Academic Press, New York.

Protocol 5.1

Determination of the concentration of viable cells in a suspension by hemocytometer counting

Materials

Phosphate buffered saline (0.1 M NaCl, 8.5 mM KCl, 0.13 M Na_2HPO_4, 1.7 mM KH_2PO_4, pH 7.4).

Trypan blue reagent: 0.2% w/v trypan blue in phosphate buffered saline.

Method

1. Add an equal volume of trypan blue reagent to a cell suspension and leave for 2 min at room temperature.

2. Apply a sample into the hemocytometer chamber by a Pasteur pipette.

3. Count cells on each of five grid blocks defined by triple lines in the hemocytometer chamber.

4. Determine the cell concentration (cells/ml) in the original sample = (2 × total count/5) × 10^4 (the calculation is based upon the volume of each grid block = 0.1 μl). The percentage of cells that are not stained with trypan blue is a measure of the viability.

Notes

1. The hemocytometer counting method is the most commonly used assay for cell viability.

2. The method is simple and effective but can be laborious for multiple samples.

3. At least 100 cells should be counted for statistical validity of the final value.

Protocol 5.2

Determination of the nuclei concentration in a culture sample

Materials

Crystal violet reagent: 0.1% w/v crystal violet in 0.1 M citric acid.

Method

1. Allow microcarriers from a culture sample (1 ml) to settle to the bottom of a centrifuge tube.

2. Remove clear supernatant by aspiration.

3. Add 1 ml of crystal violet reagent.

4. Incubate at 37°C for at least 1 h.

5. Introduce a sample into the hemocytometer chamber and count the purple-stained nuclei as for whole cells.

Notes

This method can be used to determine the nuclei concentration of anchorage-dependent cells attached to microcarriers. Care must be taken in interpreting nuclei counts as cells can become binucleated, particularly when growth is arrested. As a result the nuclei concentration may be higher than the cell concentration (Berry *et al.*, 1996).

Protocol 5.3

Determination of cell concentration by a Coulter counter

Materials

Saline solution – 0.7% NaCl, 1.05% citric acid, 0.1% mercuric chloride in distilled water.

Method

1. Add 0.5 ml of a cell suspension (10^5–10^6 cells/ml) to 19.5 ml of the saline solution.

2. Introduce the suspension into a Coulter counter (Coulter Electronics Ltd., Northwell Drive, Luton, Bedfordshire LU3 3RH, UK or 590 W. 20th Street, Hialeah, Florida 33010, USA).

3. From standard settings of the counter 0.5 ml of the suspension is counted. Multiply this count by 40 to give the original cell concentration.

Notes

1. The major advantage of the Coulter counter method is the speed of analysis and it is therefore suitable for counting a large number of samples.

2. The method is based upon the number of particles contained in suspension and, consequently, the proportion of viable cells in the sample cannot be determined.

3. It must be ensured that cell aggregates are not present in the sample; otherwise the cell count will be underestimated.

4. The Coulter counter can also be used to determine the size distribution of a cell population by careful control of the threshold settings of the instrument.

Protocol 5.4

Determination of the protein concentration of a cell suspension

---

Materials

Bradford's reagent: Dissolve 100 mg of Coomassie brilliant blue G (Sigma Chemical Co.) in 95% ethanol (50 ml) and 85% phosphoric acid (100 ml). After the dye dissolves make the solution up to 1 liter with distilled water. Alternatively, a dye (Coomassie) reagent liquid concentrate can be purchased from Biorad.

Method

1. Homogenize or sonicate a cell suspension (10^6 cells/ml).

2. Add 5 ml Bradford's reagent to 100 µl of the lysed cell sample (0–0.5 mg/ml protein).

3. Incubate for 10 min at room temperature.

4. Measure the absorbance at 595 nm.

5. Determine the sample concentrations from a standard curve, which is established from standard solutions of bovine serum albumin (BSA) at 0–0.5 mg/ml protein.

Protocol 5.5

Determination of the DNA concentration of a cell suspension

(a) Hoechst method
Materials

Buffer: 0.05 M $NaPO_4$, 2.0 M NaCl, 2 mM EDTA pH 7.4.

Hoechst reagent: 0.1 μg/ml Hoechst 33258 in buffer.

Standard DNA solution: 8 mg/ml of calf thymus DNA (Sigma Chemical Co.) in distilled water.

Method

1. Homogenize or sonicate to lyse a cell suspension (10^5 cells/ml) in buffer.

2. Dilute lysate or standard DNA solution 1 in 10 in Hoechst reagent.

3. Measure fluorescence with an excitation λ of 356 nm and emission λ of 492 nm.

4. Determine DNA concentration by reference to standard DNA.

(b) DAPI method
Materials

Buffer: 5 mM HEPES, 10 mM NaCl pH 7.

DAPI reagent: A stock solution (×100) contains 300 mg DAPI (4′,6-diamidino-2-phenylindole) in buffer.

Standard DNA solution: 8 mg/ml of calf thymus DNA (Sigma Chemical Co.) in distilled water.

Method

1. Homogenize or sonicate to lyse a cell suspension (10^5 cells/ml).

2. Dilute 150 μl lysed cell suspension with 850 μl buffer.

3. Prepare a DAPI solution (×10) by diluting 100 μl of DAPI stock solution with 900 μl of buffer and mix well. Prepare a DAPI working solution by adding 0.5 ml of DAPI (×10) to 4.5 ml of buffer.

4. Add 50 μl of DAPI working solution to each cell suspension or standard DNA (up to 0.8 μg) in a tube which is kept dark by a foil cover.

5.   Vortex the tubes and let stand for 30 min.

6.   Measure fluorescence with an excitation λ of 372 nm and emission λ of 454 nm.

7.   Determine DNA concentration by reference to the standard DNA.

Notes

1.   The DNA content of diploid cells is usually constant, although variations can occur as a result of the distribution of cells through the cell cycle. Cells in the G1 phase have the normal diploid content of DNA, which is typically 6 pg per cell.

2.   DNA measurement is probably one of the best indicators of cell concentration in solid tissue (Kurtz and Wells, 1979).

Protocol 5.6

Determination of the glucose concentration in culture

(a) Glucose oxidase assay

Materials

Glucose oxidase/peroxidase reagent. Dissolve the contents of a reagent capsule from Sigma in 39.2 ml of distilled water. Each capsule contains 500 units of glucose oxidase and 100 units of peroxidase.

O-Dianisidine reagent. Dissolve the contents of a vial of o-dianisidine (Sigma Chemical Co.) in 1 ml of distilled water. Each vial contains 5 mg of o-dianisidine dihydrochloride.

Assay reagent. Mix 0.8 ml of o-dianisidine reagent with 39.2 ml of glucose oxidase/peroxidase reagent.

Glucose standard solution. 1 mg/ml of D-glucose.

Sulfuric acid, 12 M.

Method

1. Start the reaction by adding 2 ml of assay reagent to glucose standard or culture media supernatant (0.01–0.1 ml). Make the assay volume up to 3 ml with distilled water.

2. Allow the reaction to proceed for 30 min at 37°C.

3. Stop the reaction by adding 2 ml of 12 M H_2SO_4.

4. Measure the absorbance at 540 nm.

5. Determine the glucose concentration of the media samples against standard values obtained with the glucose solution.

Notes

Reaction 1 is catalyzed by glucose oxidase (GOD) and reaction 2 by peroxidase (POD). The dye, o-dianisidine hydrochloride is reduced by hydrogen peroxide to a product which has a pink color in the presence of sulfuric acid (reaction 3) and is measured colorimetrically. The glucose oxidase kit from Sigma Chemical Co. contains glucose oxidase/peroxidase reagent and o-dianisidine reagent.

D-glucose + H_2O + O_2 → D-gluconic acid + H_2O_2 (1)

H_2O_2 + reduced o-dianisidine →$2H_2O$ + oxidized o-dianisidine (brown)   (2)

oxidized o-dianisidine (brown) + H_2SO_4 → oxidized o-dianisidine (pink)   (3)

(Bergmeyer and Bernt, 1974).

(b) Hexokinase assay
Materials

Glucose (HK) assay reagent. Dissolve the contents of a reagent vial (Sigma) into 20 ml of distilled water. The dissolved reagent contains 1.5 mM NAD, 1.0 mM ATP, 1 unit/ml hexokinase and 1 unit/ml glucose 6-phosphate dehydrogenase.

Glucose standard solution. 1 mg/ml of D-glucose.

Method

1. Mix 10–200 μl of standard glucose solution or sample of culture media with 1 ml of assay reagent. Make the total assay volume up to 2 ml with distilled water.

2. Incubate at room temperature for 15 min.

3. Measure the absorbance at 340 nm.

4. Determine the glucose concentration of the media samples against standard values obtained with the glucose solution.

Notes

Hexokinase converts glucose into glucose 6-phosphate (G-6P) in the presence of ATP (reaction 1). The G-6P is immediately converted into 6-phosphogluconate by glucose 6-phosphate dehydrogenase (reaction 2). The associated formation of NADH is monitored by the change in absorbance at 340 nm and this is proportional to the concentration of glucose originally present. The hexokinase kit from Sigma Chemical Co. contains a hexokinase/glucose 6-phosphate dehydrogenase reagent. The kit includes a glucose standard solution (1 mg/ml).

$$\text{D-glucose} + \text{ATP} \rightarrow \text{glucose-6P} + \text{ADP} \qquad (1)$$
$$\text{glucose-6P} + \text{NAD} \rightarrow \text{6-phosphogluconate} + \text{NADH} + \text{H}^+ \qquad (2)$$

The sensitivity of this assay can be increased by measuring the rate of increase of absorbance at 340 nm. This can be achieved with a recording spectrophotometer or using the kinetic mode of a multi-well plate reader (Kunst et al., 1984).

(c) The glucose analyzer
Equipment

YSI model 27 Industrial Analyzer (Yellow Spring Instrument Co., Inc., Yellow Springs, Ohio 45387, USA).

Method

1. Fit the appropriate membrane into the analyzer for glucose analysis.

2. Calibrate the instrument with standard glucose solutions (2–5 g/l).

3.   Inject 25 μl of a cell-free sample of culture supernatant into the instrument and compare with standard readings.

Notes

1.   The sample is injected into a membrane which converts the glucose to hydrogen peroxide which can be determined by a sensor system based on a Clark electrode. The latter consists of a platinum electrode which measures the hydrogen peroxide amperometrically.

$$H_2O_2 \rightarrow 2H^+ + O_2 + 2e- \tag{1}$$

$$AgCl + e- \rightarrow Ag + Cl- \tag{2}$$

Current flow in the platinum anode is linearly proportional to the local concentration of hydrogen peroxide. This electrode is maintained at an electrical potential of 0.7 V with respect to a silver/silver chloride reference electrode, the potential of which is determined by the reaction above. The signal current which is proportional to the quantity of injected glucose is converted to a voltage by the instrument circuitry.

2.   This method of analysis is particularly suitable for the analysis of glucose in multiple samples of culture medium.

3.   By the selection of the appropriate membrane in this instrument various analytes can be determined such as glucose, sucrose, starch, lactose, galactose, glycerin, lactate or ethanol.

Protocol 5.7

Determination of the viable concentration of cells by dye exclusion: the tetrazolium assay

Materials

MTT reagent: 5 mg/ml of the tetrazolium dye (Sigma Chemical Co.), MTT (3-(4,5-dimethylthiazol-2-yl)-2,5-diphenyltetrazolium bromide) in phosphate buffered saline (PBS) pH 7.4.

SDS reagent: 10% w/v sodium dodecyl sulfate (SDS), 45% w/v N,N-dimethyl formamide in water adjusted to pH 4.5 with glacial acetic acid.

Method

1. Remove the media from adherent cells in a multi-well plate and add 0.1 ml MTT reagent. Alternatively, add 0.1 ml MTT reagent to a 1 ml cell suspension in PBS.

2. Incubate for 2 h at 37°C.

3. Add 600 µl of SDS reagent and mix to solubilize the formazan crystals.

4. Measure the absorbance at 570 nm.

Notes

1. The method is particularly convenient for the rapid assay of replicate cell cultures in multi-well plates. Plate readers are capable of measuring the absorbance of each well of a standard 96-well plate.

2. It is important to ensure that the colored formazan salt formed from MTT is completely dissolved in the SDS reagent.

3. Alternatively, tetrazolium salts can be used in this assay such as XTT and WST-1 which are available from Boehringer-Mannheim. These form soluble colored products.

Protocol 5.8

Determination of cell viability by lactate dehydrogenase determination

Method

1. Mix 2.8 ml Tris HCl (0.2 M) pH 7.3, 0.1 ml NADH (6.6 mM) and 0.1 ml sodium pyruvate (30 mM) in a cuvette.

2. Pre-incubate for 5 min at the desired reaction temperature (25°C or 37°C).

3. Start reaction by adding 50 μl of sample or standard LDH enzyme (Sigma Chemical Co.).

4. Record enzyme activity as an absorbance decrease at 340 nm.

Notes

1. This method is well suited for the determination of multiple samples, particularly if a multi-well plate reader is available.

2. Care must be taken when interpreting the results by this method because the LDH content per cell can change considerably during the course of batch culture.

3. The loss of cell viability can be expressed as the activity of LDH in the medium as a proportion of total LDH in the culture.

Protocol 5.9

Determination of the intracellular energy charge

_____

Materials

ATP monitoring reagent/ATP-MR (LKB/BioOrbit, PO Box 36, 20521 Turku, 52 Finland) contains a lyophilized mixture of firefly luciferase, D-luciferin, bovine serum albumin, magnesium acetate and inorganic pyrophosphate. Re-constitute each vial with 4 ml buffer plus 1 ml potassium acetate (1 M).

ATP standards (LKB): ATP (0.1 µmol) and magnesium sulfate (2 µmol).

Buffer: 0.1 M Tris-acetate pH 7.75.

PK-PEP reagent: 55 µl tricyclohexylammonium salt of phosphoenolpyruvate (0.2 M) + 50 µl pyruvate kinase (500 U/mg) in Tris buffer.

MK-CTP reagent: 95 µl myokinase (2500 U/mg) + 10 µl CTP (110 mM) in Tris buffer.

Method

1. Extract soluble nucleotides by addition of 0.1 ml perchloric acid (20% v/v) to 1 ml of a cell culture sample (10^6 cells/ml).

2. Place on ice for 15 min and centrifuge for 5 min at 10 000 *g*.

3. Remove supernatant and neutralize with 5 M KOH.

4. For ATP determination: Mix 860 µl buffer, 100 µl ATP-MR and 10 µl sample.

5. For ADP determination: Add a further 10 µl PK-PEP.

6. For AMP determination: Add a further 10 µl MK-CTP.

7. For standardization: Add a further 10 µl ATP standard.

8. Measure the light emission in a luminometer (for example, LKB 1250) after 1 min of each stage of addition.

Notes

1. The luminescence assay is dependent upon the emission of light resulting from the enzymic oxidation of luciferin, a reaction requiring ATP.

    $$ATP + LH_2 + O_2 \rightarrow AMP + PPi + CO_2 + L + light$$

2. ADP and AMP can also be measured by the luciferase assay after conversion to ATP by coupled enzymic reactions.

Pyruvate kinase:

ADP + PEP → ATP + pyruvate

Myokinase:

AMP + CTP → ADP + CDP

3. The measurement of energy charge is more time consuming than the routine counting procedures discussed earlier but can allow a means of monitoring the decline in the energy metabolism of a cell culture that occurs during the loss of viability (Lundin *et al.*, 1986).

Protocol 5.10

Determination of the cellular rate of protein synthesis

Method

1. Add ^{3}H-leucine or ^{35}S-methionine (Amersham) at a final specific activity of 20–40 µCi/ml to cell suspension at 5–10 $\times$ 10^6 cells/ml.

2. Remove 5–10 $\times$ 10^5 cells at each time point up to 4–6 h.

3. Isolate cell pellet by centrifugation in a microcentrifuge tube and wash in PBS.

4. Precipitate protein by addition of 500 µl trichloroacetic acid/TCAA (5%) containing unlabeled amino acids.

5. Wash the protein precipitate three times in the TCAA solution.

6. Add 30 µl NCS™ tissue solubilizer (Amersham) to the pellet and leave for 60 min.

7. Cut tip of tube and place in scintillation fluid for radioactive counting.

Notes

1. The cells should be incubated in the medium for sufficient time to measure radioactivity in the extracted cell pellet. Normally 4–6 h is sufficient but this may be longer.

2. The rate of DNA synthesis of a cell population can be determined in a similar assay to that described for protein synthesis but using a radioactively labeled nucleotide precursor such as tritiated thymidine (^{3}H-TdR) or deoxycytidine (^{3}H-CdR; Amersham).

3. The exposure period may be short (30–60 min) for DNA synthesis rate determinations and a specific activity of 1 µCi/ml of culture is sufficient.

4. Higher specific activities may be required if using culture media containing the corresponding nonradioactive components such as methionine or thymidine.

Protocol 5.11

Cell characterization by Giemsa banding of chromosomes (karyotype analysis)

Materials

Colcemid (20 μg/ml).

Hypotonic solution (0.075 M KCl).

Fixative solution (methanol/acetic acid 3:1 v/v).

Staining solution (6.5 ml PBS, 0.5 ml trypsin 1%, 2.5 ml methanol and 0.22 ml Giemsa).

Method

1. Add colcemid (final concentration: 0.1–0.4 μg/ml) to a T-flask containing cells growing in exponential phase.

2. Remove the medium after approximately 6 h. For attached cells this can be by decanting.

3. Collect cells by centrifugation (for suspension cells) or by trypsinization and centrifugation (attached cells).

4. Allow the cells to swell in a hypotonic solution (0.075 M KCl) for 15 min at 37 °C.

5. Collect cells by centrifugation, re-suspend in 0.075 M KCl and slowly add the fixative solution. Leave for 20 min.

6. Collect cells and re-suspend in the fixative.

7. Add the cell suspension dropwise onto a microscope slide and allow to dry.

8. Flood the slide with trypsin–Giemsa staining solution and leave for 15 min.

9. Observe the stained chromosome spreads microscopically. A photomicrograph will allow close inspection and analysis of the individual chromosomes.

Notes

1. Colcemid is a mitotic inhibitor and will block cells at mitosis. At this stage distinct chromosomes can be seen in the nuclei of cells.

2. The hypotonic solution causes cell swelling and maximizes separation between chromosomes.

3. The staining solution containing trypsin and Giemsa will break down associated protein and will stain the chromosomes with a characteristic pattern of G-bands.

Chapter 6

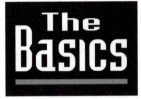

Genetic engineering of animal cells in culture

1. Introduction

The discovery of methods to isolate and transfer DNA from one species to another has led to numerous advances in understanding the function and regulatory mechanisms of individual genes. The technology has also been applied to genetically manipulate cells so that they become capable of expressing high levels of a selected protein ('overexpression'). This usually follows the transfer of a recombinant DNA incorporated into a vector that ensures rates of transcription and subsequent expression of the recombinant protein (*Figure 6.1*). The techniques could be the basis of designing experiments aimed at explaining the control of protein synthesis or cell differentiation. This is also the basis of large-scale production of the protein products of selected human genes. In this chapter, we will consider some of these

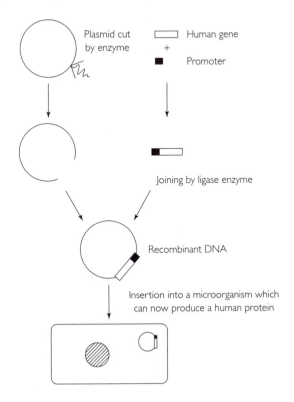

Figure 6.1

Transfection of a human gene into a cell with a plasmid.

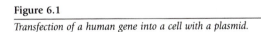

techniques in relation to animal cell cultures. These possibilities have led to the increased commercial activity and interest in animal cell technology over the last 10 years.

2. The need for mammalian cells

Mammalian cells have been the host cells of choice for the synthesis of complex glycoproteins from recombinant genes. They have the required characteristics for appropriate post-translational processing and product secretion. The most widely used host cell line for recombinant DNA has been the Chinese Hamster Ovary (CHO). The metabolism of this cell has been well studied and characterized. A number of vectors have been designed to provide high yields of a range of biologically active mammalian proteins from these cells.

3. How to get DNA into mammalian cells

Transfection means the transfer of nucleic acid into mammalian cells although it can also be referred to as DNA-mediated transformation. This should not be confused with the alternative use of 'transformation' meaning a change of growth characteristics of animal cells from a finite to an indefinite lifespan (see Chapter 2). The ability of mammalian cells to incorporate foreign DNA was first shown in the early 1960s when mutant human cells which lacked the enzyme hypoxanthine-guanine phosphoribosyl transferase (HGPRT) were transfected with isolated human nuclear DNA (Szybalska and Szybalska, 1962). Transfected cells were subsequently found with a functional gene for the HGPRT enzyme (see Chapter 8).

A variety of methods is now available for incorporating foreign DNA into animal cells. However, this does not always lead to the expression of a corresponding protein. Protein expression is dependent upon the incorporation of a structural gene along with the required expression signals into the cell (see Section 5).

Here, we will consider some of the methods that can be used to introduce the DNA into the cells. One important criterion for choosing a particular method is that the yield of transfected cells is sufficiently high to allow easy isolation. Also, some methods are better than others in allowing the foreign DNA to integrate with the cell's nuclear DNA and allowing stable expression of protein.

3.1 Transfer of 'naked' DNA

■ Calcium phosphate method. DNA uptake into cells can be aided by co-precipitation of DNA with calcium phosphate (Wigler et al., 1979). The precipitate is adsorbed onto the cell membrane before being incorporated into the cells, a process enhanced by brief exposure to dimethyl sulfoxide (DMSO) or to glycerol. By this method, the proportion of cells taking up the DNA precipitate is high. However, the proportion of the cells that take up the precipitate into the nucleus is relatively low (1–2%). Gene expression will occur in a small proportion of these cells and an even smaller proportion will be stably transfected. This method has been used extensively as a general and simple method for introducing DNA into mammalian cells.

- DEAE-dextran. Transfection of cells by DNA complexed to the polymer, diethylaminoethyl dextran can be successful, particularly if accompanied by treatment with DMSO, which causes temporary destabilization of the cell membrane. A high proportion of a cell population can be transfected by this method but this generally leads only to transient protein expression.

- Encapsulation of DNA in liposome vesicles is an effective way to improve the efficiency of cellular uptake. The liposomes are complexes formed from a positively charged lipid and DNA. The complexes are readily taken up by mammalian cells. A suitable cationic lipid reagent is Lipofectamine, which is a proprietary formulation supplied by Invitrogen. The reagent is complexed with DNA or RNA prior to transfection of a suspension of preconfluent cells. The procedure allows rapid high-efficiency transfections that result in high levels of gene expression. (*Protocol 6.1.*)

- Electroporation involves the exposure of a cell suspension to a high-voltage electrical impulse. Transient pores that are formed in the cell membrane promote the uptake of DNA. The conditions for electroporation are determined experimentally so as to maximize the number of surviving transfected cells. Typically, the cells are subjected to electrical impulses of 100–200 V for 1–2 ms. (*Protocol 6.2.*)

- Micro-injection involves the insertion of DNA by a micro-needle into the nucleus of individual cells. This is an effective technique for inserting DNA into a small number of cells but is generally only performed by a specialized laboratory. 'Hits' are almost certain but the technique cannot be applied to a large number of cells.

- Protoplast fusion. Plasmids which are grown in bacteria can be introduced directly into animal cells by cell fusion with the bacterial protoplast. The protoplast is prepared by lysozyme treatment of the bacteria to remove the cell wall. The bacterial protoplast is fused to a mammalian cell by treatment with polyethylene glycol. The entire content of the bacterial cell is introduced into the mammalian cell and this has the advantage of not requiring DNA purification. However, difficulties can arise from the introduction of unwanted bacterial components into the recipient cells.

3.2   DNA transfer using viruses

Viruses are efficient vectors for DNA transfer – a process termed transduction. Animal viruses have important characteristics that increase the efficiency of nucleic acid transfer into mammalian cells:

- they promote the transfer of DNA to cells because of capsid proteins that bind to cell membrane receptors;
- they contain promoters that allow expression of inserted genes in animal cells;
- they replicate to high copy numbers, that is produce several copies of the required gene within each cell;
- some viruses integrate efficiently into the animal cell genome.

The most widely used viral expression system has been derived from a simian virus, SV40 (Rigby, 1982). The virus contains a circular DNA duplex of 5.2 kilobases and many well-characterized sites of cleavage by restriction endonucleases. During SV40 infection of mammalian cells there are two phases of transcription. In the early phase, proteins known as the 'T antigens' are synthesized. This causes unwinding of the viral DNA leading to the late-phase transcription and production of the viral capsid proteins. The infectious cycle takes about 70 hours and eventually leads to cell lysis.

In recombinant virus vectors, part of the viral genome is replaced by foreign DNA. These can be constructed as early or late region replacement vectors. The advantage of this type of vector is that DNA is introduced into the cell by viral infection – a process which is extremely efficient. However, the system has a limited host range (only monkey cells) and is suitable only for small foreign DNA inserts. The potential size of the foreign DNA insert can be increased if only a small portion of the SV40 DNA is utilized, such as the promoter region. This has been used extensively as a transient expression system (see Section 5.1).

Efficient vectors for integration of foreign genes into animal cells have been developed from retroviruses (Cepko *et al.*, 1984). Retroviruses can integrate genes into the nuclear DNA. These viruses have an RNA genome which requires the formation of complementary DNA copies by the enzyme reverse transcriptase. In the normal process of infection, the DNA can be integrated into the host cell's genome without causing cell lysis. The retroviruses can be used for cell immortalization (see Chapter 2).

Recombinant vectors are constructed by replacement of the retroviral structural genes with foreign DNA. They have the ability to replicate and integrate into the host cell's DNA but not for forming viral coat proteins.

Table 6.1 shows a summary of the advantages and disadvantages of using the alternative methods of transfection discussed in this section.

Table 6.1. Advantages and disadvantages of methods of introducing DNA into cultured animal cells

Method	Advantage	Disadvantage
Calcium phosphate	Simple	Low incorporation into nucleus
DEAE-dextran	Simple	Transient expression only
Liposomes	Simple	Relatively unproven
Electroporation	Good for nonadherent cells	No cotransfection
Micro-injection	Efficient	Efficient/technically difficult
Protoplast fusion	Good for nonadherent cells	Variable results
SV40 virus infection	Efficient	Cell-type restricted
Retrovirus infection	Efficient	Cell-type restricted

Adapted from MacDonald, C. (1991) Genetic engineering of animal cells. In: Butler, M. (ed.) *Mammalian Cell Biotechnology: A Practical Approach*, pp. 57–83. Oxford University Press, Oxford.

4. How to select and amplify the genes of transfected cells

4.1 Cell selection by genetic markers

The proportion of cells that accept exogenous DNA during a transfection process may be as low as 1 in 10^6 and therefore a means of selection of the transfected cells is essential. To allow selection, a marker gene can be incorporated into a recipient cell. The purpose of the genetic marker is to identify the cells that have been transfected . The marker can be linked to the same DNA vector as the target gene. However, direct ligation of the two genes may not be necessary because of the phenomenon of cotransfection. This follows the observation that more than one gene can be transfected into a cell at the same time even if they are located on separate plasmids. This is explained by the fact that although only a few cells take up exogenous DNA, the recipient cells accept relatively large amounts of DNA.

Gene markers that have been used extensively in mammalian cells include genes for the enzymes hypoxanthine guanine phosphoribosyl transferase (HGPRT), thymidine kinase (TK) and dihydrofolate reductase (DHFR). These are nondominant marker genes and can only be used for selection in a population of cells that are mutants, lacking the marker enzyme activity prior to transfection (see Chapter 8, Section 6.4).

Dominant genes are more useful because they do not require mutant recipient cells and can be used with any cell type. One example is the gene for the enzyme xanthine-guanine phosphoribosyl transferase (XGPRT) which is only present in bacteria and permits the metabolism of xanthine (*Figure 6.2*). Only recipient mammalian cells that have acquired the bacterial gene during transfection can survive in a medium containing xanthine, hypoxanthine and mycophenolic acid, which inhibits the conversion of IMP to XMP. Selection can be improved by the addition of aminopterin which

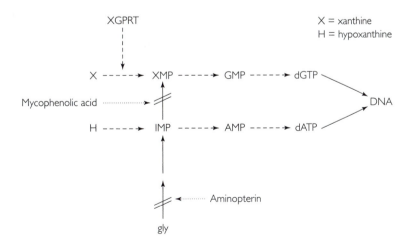

Figure 6.2

The effect of the XGPRT selection system on purine metabolism.

inhibits *de novo* nucleotide synthesis, making the cells entirely dependent upon the bacterial enzyme for purine nucleotide synthesis.

Antibiotic resistance genes are also suitable as dominant markers. For example, the neomycin-resistance gene (neo^R) codes for the enzyme amino-glycoside phosphotransferase. The presence of this enzyme confers resistance to the aminoglycoside group of antibiotics of which G418 is the one most commonly used. G418 prevents replication of mammalian cells. If the neo^R gene is expressed then the cells survive.

4.2   Gene amplification

This involves an increase in the number of copies of a specific gene per cell and can result in increased synthesis of the corresponding protein. Gene amplification was first demonstrated in mammalian cells by selection for resistance to methotrexate which is an analog of folic acid and competitive inhibitor of the dihydrofolate reductase enzyme, DHFR (Alt *et al.*, 1978). This enzyme is essential for the conversion of the folate co-enzyme required in purine and pyrimidine metabolism (*Figure 6.3a*). Cellular resistance to the effects of methotrexate can occur by a stepwise increase in the concentration of methotrexate in the culture medium (*Protocol 6.3*). Cells that become resistant to methotrexate fall into one of three classes: (a) reduced methotrexate uptake; (b) point mutation in the dhfr gene making the enzyme less susceptible to inhibition; and (c) multiple copies of the dhfr locus allowing the production of sufficient enzyme to compete with the effect of the inhibitor. In the third class, resistance is brought about by the amplification of the gene for dihydrofolate reductase (DHFR). These resistant cells are selected by successive increases in the dosage of methotrexate. The cells can have highly amplified dhfr gene arrays, allowing the growth of cells in concentrations of methotrexate up to $\times 10^5$ the dose lethal to nonresistant wild-type cells. It is important to realize that methotrexate does not induce gene amplification, rather it provides selective pressure for the isolation of cells that have undergone random gene amplification.

The gene amplification is stable and results in corresponding increases in the enzyme levels in the cell. Co-amplification of an associated gene will occur if the gene is inserted adjacent to the DHFR gene on the vector. By this

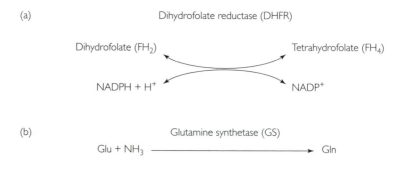

(a)   Dihydrofolate reductase (DHFR)

Dihydrofolate (FH$_2$)   Tetrahydrofolate (FH$_4$)

NADPH + H$^+$ NADP$^+$

(b)   Glutamine synthetase (GS)

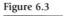   Glu + NH$_3$ 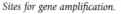 Gln

Figure 6.3

Sites for gene amplification.

method stable cell lines can be produced with as much as a 1000-fold increase in gene copy number and corresponding protein expression.

An alternative system involves the gene for glutamine synthetase which is amplified by addition of methionine sulfoximine (Bebbington *et al.*, 1992). The enzyme is required for the conversion of glutamate to glutamine which is essential for the growth of cells in the absence of glutamine (*Figure 6.3b*).

5. How to get genes to express proteins

The insertion of DNA into a cell does not guarantee gene expression and synthesis of the corresponding protein. DNA transcription requires a number of expression signals which are specific for mammalian cells. The expression signals are usually added to the gene before it is transfected into a cell and is referred to as an 'expression system'. Various ways have been devised to increase the chances of the expression of proteins by isolated mammalian genes (Hentschel, 1991). The efficiencies of expression vary and depend upon the gene, expression signals and the cell line used.

Stable gene expression is dependent upon the integration of a segment of DNA into the nucleus of the host cell line or an efficient extrachromosomal replication system that is maintained during cell division. Depending upon the method used, gene expression may be transient or stable.

5.1 Transient gene expression

This is generally used as a preliminary test of gene expression. The production of a protein from a transfected cell is assayed from a sample of the cell culture after a short period of time – usually 1–3 days following the uptake of DNA. For this, the transfected cells need not be selected or isolated but the rate of incorporation and expression of DNA in the cells needs to be high. However, the cells are not genetically stable and soon lose their expression ability.

The most commonly used transient expression system involves COS cells (Gluzman, 1981). These are monkey kidney cells transfected with a mutant SV40 virus having an inactivated origin of DNA replication (six basepair deletion). The SV40 DNA is not replicated because of this deletion. However, any transfected DNA containing a functional SV40 origin of replication can be replicated in these cells. A suitable vector contains the small SV40 DNA fragment as well as any cloned gene of interest. These can be transfected into COS cells to obtain high copy numbers of the cloned gene ($2–5 \times 10^5$ copies/cell). However, permanent cell lines can not be established by this method because the extensive viral replication eventually has an adverse effect on the viability of the cells.

5.2 Stable gene expression

Stable expression systems are used to construct and isolate transfected cells that are genetically stable and are capable of indefinite synthesis of a particular protein. Recombinant vectors can be constructed that maximize the chances of obtaining such cells. The limiting factor in obtaining stable transfected cells is usually the frequency of DNA integration, rather than the frequency of cellular uptake. The ideal recombinant cell is one that grows with a doubling time of ~18 h, is genetically stable and secretes a recombinant protein at ~20% of total cellular protein.

The most commonly used cell line for the stable expression of a recombinant protein is the Chinese hamster ovary (CHO) line – primarily because the cells have been well studied and characterized. Vectors are constructed with a variety of domains to ensure efficient, high-level expression of the desired protein in mammalian cells. Many of these vectors have nucleotide sequences from the bacteria plasmid pBR322. This enables vector replication in bacteria or mammalian cells (termed a shuttle vector).

5.3   Expression cassettes

A number of expression signals are needed to ensure that a gene is expressed in mammalian cells. These signals are common to a wide variety of genes and can be used in a range of cell lines. An expression cassette is a DNA sequence containing these signal sequences that is incorporated into a vector used to transfect mammalian cells. The signal sequences of an expression cassette include the following.

- A promoter that is required to initiate transcription of the gene. This marks the point at which transcription of a gene starts following RNA polymerase binding. Promoters contain highly conserved sequences (for example, the 'TATA' box or 'initiator') located upstream of the initial site of transcription. Promoters taken from an animal virus (for example, SV40, adeno- or retroviruses) have been used to express a number of transfected genes. These are described as 'strong promoters' because they allow a high rate of transcription.
- A ribosome-binding site is a short nucleotide sequence required for attachment of mRNA to ribosomes.
- A terminator is required downstream of the expressed gene to mark the point at which transcription stops.

Figure 6.4 shows the elements of a shuttle vector which contains an expression cassette. This recombinant vector, named SVX, contains the following elements:

- promoter and termination control regions from a retrovirus;
- the mammalian gene inserted for expression – in this example (*Figure 6.4*) globin cDNA is inserted;
- a selectable marker gene for neomycin (neo) resistance (see Section 4.1);
- origin of replication sites (ori) enabling replication in either bacteria or mammalian cells.

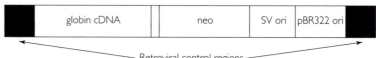

Figure 6.4

Shuttle vector construct, SVX.

6. Regulation of gene expression

The ability to regulate the expression of a foreign gene by the addition of an external stimulus can have distinct advantages. In some cases, overexpression of a specific protein can be growth inhibitory or toxic to cells. So, it would be an advantage to switch off gene expression during cell growth and only allow the foreign gene to be expressed when maximum cell density is attained.

This type of switching mechanism requires a regulated promoter such as the one isolated from mouse mammary tumor virus, which can be induced by dexamethasone. The inducible promoter can be used to induce the transcription of any gene associated with it in an expression vector when dexamethasone is added to the culture medium. The presence of the promoter can also enhance the level of protein expression (Klessig *et al.*, 1984).

References

Alt, F.W., Kellems, R.E., Bertino, J.R. and Schimke, R.T. (1978) Selective multiplication of dihydrofolate reductase genes in methotrexate-resistant variants of cultured murine cells. *J. Biol. Chem.* **253**: 1357–1370.

Bebbington, C.R., Renner, G., Thomson, S., King, D., Abrams, D. and Yarranton, G.T. (1992) Recombinant antibody from myeloma cells using a glutamine synthetase gene as an amplifiable selective marker. *Biotechnology* **10**: 169–175.

Cepko, C., Roberts, B.E. and Mulligan, R.C. (1984) Construction and applications of a highly transmissible retrovirus shuttle vector. *Cell* **37**: 1053–1062.

Gluzman, Y. (1981) SV40–transformed simian cells support the replication of early SV40 mutants. *Cell* **23**: 175–182.

Hentschel, C.C. (1991) Recent developments in mammalian expression systems. In: Spier, R.E., Griffiths, J.B. and Meigner, B. *et al.* (eds) *Production of Biologicals from Animal Cells in Culture*, pp. 287–303. Butterworth, Oxford.

Klessig, D.F., Brough, D.E. and Cleghon, V. (1984) Introduction, stable integration and controlled expression of a chimeric adenovirus gene whose product is toxic to the recipient human cell. *Molec. Cell Biol.* **4**: 1354–1362.

MacDonald, C. (1991) Genetic engineering of animal cells. In: Butler, M. (ed.) *Mammalian Cell Biotechnology: A Practical Approach*, pp. 57–83. Oxford University Press, Oxford.

Rigby, P.W.J. (1982) Expression of cloned genes in eukaryotic cells using vector systems derived from viral replicons. In: Williamson, R. (ed.) *Genetic Engineering*, Vol. 3, pp. 83–141. Academic Press, London.

Szybalska, E.H. and Szybalska, W. (1962) Genetics of human cell lines, IV. DNA-mediated heritable transformation of a biochemical trait. *Proc. Natl Acad. Sci.* **48**: 2026–2034.

Wigler, M., Sweet, R., Sim, G.K., Wold, B., Pellicer, A., Lacy, E., Maniatis, T., Silverstein, S. and Axel, R. (1979) Transformation of mammalian cells with genes from procaryotes and eucaryotes. *Cell* **16**: 777–785.

Further reading

Brown, T.A. (2001) *Gene Cloning and DNA Analysis*. Blackwell Science, Oxford.

Glover, D.M. (ed.) (1987) *DNA Cloning: A Practical Approach*, Vol.1–3. IRL Press, Oxford.

Hardin, C.C., Edwards, J., Robertson, D. and Miller, W. (eds) (2001) *Cloning, Gene Expression and Protein Purification. Experimental Procedures and Process Rationale*. Oxford University Press, Oxford.

Heiser, W.C. (2004) *Gene Delivery to Mammalian Cells: Methods and Protocols (Methods in Molecular Biology)*. Humana Press, New Jersey.

Howe, C. (1995) *Gene Cloning and Manipulation*. Cambridge University Press, Cambridge.

Jones, P. (ed.) (1998) *Vectors: Cloning Applications: Essential Techniques.* J. Wiley & Sons, New Jersey.

Kaufman, R.J. (1990) Use of recombinant DNA technology for engineering mammalian cells to produce proteins. In: Lubiniecki, A.S. (ed.) *Large-Scale Mammalian Cell Culture Technology*, pp.15–69. Marcel Dekker, New York.

Kingsman, S.M. and Kingsman, A.J. (1988) *Genetic Engineering: An Introduction to Gene Analysis and Exploitation in Eukaryotes.* Blackwell, Oxford.

Old, R.W. and Primrose, S.B. (1989) *Principles of Gene Manipulation: An Introduction to Genetic Engineering.* Blackwell, Oxford.

Ravid, K. and Freshney, R.I. (eds) (1978) *DNA Transfer to Cultured Cells.* J. Wiley & Sons, New Jersey.

Sambrook, J., Fritsch, E.F. and Maniatis, T. (1989) *Molecular Cloning: A Laboratory Manual.* Cold Harbor Laboratory Press, New York.

Weymouth, L.A. and Barsoum, J. (1986) Genetic engineering in mammalian cells. pp. 9–62 In: Thilly, W.G. (ed.) *Mammalian Cell Technology.* Butterworth, Boston.

Protocol 6.1

Transfection of CHO-K1 cells by lipofection

Materials

OptiMEM 1 (Invitrogen), Lipofectamine 2000 (Invitrogen).

Method

1. Prepare cells. Incubate 1.5×10^5 cells in 0.5 ml growth medium for 24 h in each well of a 24-well plate so that the culture becomes >90% confluent.

2. Prepare the DNA–lipid complex

   - Dilute 0.8 μg DNA with 50 μl OptiMEM.

   - Dilute 2.5 μl Lipofectamine 2000 with 50 μl OptiMEM and incubate for 5 min at room temperature.

   - Combine the diluted DNA and Lipofectamine. Incubate at room temperature for 20 min to form the DNA–lipid complex.

3. Transfection

   - Add the DNA–Lipofectamine complex (100 μl) to each well of cells.

   - Mix gently by rocking the plate and incubate at 37°C for at least 24 h before testing for transgene expression.

Protocol 6.2

Transfection by electroporation

Method

1. Suspend cells in serum-free medium.

2. Add 10 µg DNA or RNA to 10^7 cells.

3. Electroporate at 688 V/cm; 800 µF using the Cell-Porator Electroporation System (Gibco BRL).

Protocol 6.3

Development and isolation of methotrexate-resistant CHO cells

---

Materials

CHO dhfr$^-$ cell culture in exponential growth.

Methotrexate in 0.15 M NaCl (2.5 mg/ml).

Method

1. Inoculate the CHO cells from an exponentially growing culture into replicate T-flasks containing 0, 0.01, 0.02, 0.05 and 0.1 μg/ml methotrexate added to the culture media from the stock solution.

2. Incubate for 5 to 7 days.

3. Replace with medium containing the same amounts of methotrexate and allow to grow for another 5 to 7 days.

4. When the cell density in each flask reaches 2–10 × 10^6 cells/flask, remove the cells and inoculate into medium containing the same and higher (×2 and ×10) concentrations of methotrexate.

5. Allow to grow for 5–7 days and select viable cells for subculture. Isolate small proportions of cells showing clonal growth in a background of enlarged or dying cells.

6. Continue selection and subculture with progressively higher methotrexate concentrations until the desired level of resistance is obtained. This can take 3–6 months for high levels of resistance.

Notes

It is important to store cell samples from subcultures periodically. This will safeguard against loss of cultures by poor growth or contamination. If cell samples are stored, then the procedure can be resumed at the previous point of methotrexate resistance.

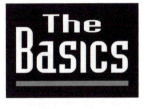

Chapter 7

The glycosylation of proteins in cell culture

1. Introduction

Most large proteins derived from animals have attached carbohydrate structures (glycans) that are added as a post-translational modification. At one time these glycans were thought to be unimportant to glycoprotein activity. However, now it is clear that an understanding of the carbohydrate component (glycan) of a recombinant glycoprotein is of importance for two main reasons. Firstly, the carbohydrate structures attached to a protein can affect many of its properties. This includes its pharmacokinetics, bioactivity, secretion, *in vivo* clearance, solubility, recognition and antigenicity, all of which influence the overall therapeutic profile of the glycoprotein. Secondly, quantitative and qualitative aspects of glycosylation can be affected by the production process in culture, including the host cell line, method of culture, extracellular environment and the protein itself (Jenkins and Curling, 1994).

Glycosylation is a process that occurs in eukaryotic cells in which oligosaccharides are added to the protein during synthesis and processed through the endoplasmic reticulum (ER) and Golgi apparatus along the secretory pathway. Glycoproteins occur as heterogeneous populations of molecules, called glycoforms (Rudd and Dwek, 1997). Glycomics is a term used for the analysis of heterogeneous pools of glycans. It is important to realize that the structure of the glycan is not governed by a predetermined template as is the case for proteins and a variety of structures are possible for any protein. The potential variability of glycoforms presents a difficulty to industrial production and for regulatory approval of therapeutic glycoproteins. The challenge is to know how the glycoprotein heterogeneity is generated, and how to evaluate its significance with respect to the safety and efficacy of the product (Jenkins *et al.*, 1996).

The glycoforms have characteristic profiles that can vary with the control parameters of bioprocessing. It is important to understand these culture control parameters to assure the reproducibility of a bioprocess to yield the same glycoform profile that went through clinical trials and to maximize the titer of the desired glycoforms.

There are several advantages in using mammalian cells for the production of recombinant glycoproteins. One of the most important of these is their ability to perform post-translational modifications and achieve a product close to that produced *in vivo*. The use of other expression systems such as yeast, plant or insect cells is more limited because despite their potential economic advantages for culture and the higher yields of these systems, their glycosylation capacities do not resemble those of the mammalian cells.

Glycosylation engineering is gaining importance as a tool to optimize desirable properties such as stability, antigenicity and bioactivity of glycosylated therapeutic pharmaceuticals. This is achieved by genetic engineering of the pathways of oligosaccharide synthesis in the mammalian host cells. Incorporation of new glycosyltransferase activities can modify the product, compete with endogenous enzymes to produce novel glycoforms or maximize the proportion of beneficial ones.

The purpose of this chapter is to outline the capabilities of various cell lines for recombinant glycoprotein production. Each cell line's capacity for glycosylation may be modified by parameters associated with growth of the cells in culture. These combined factors will lead to a heterogeneity of glycoforms that will be considered in relation to their acceptability for use as human therapeutic agents.

2.   Glycan structures present in glycoproteins

There are three types of glycan structures attached to proteins: N-glycans, O-glycans and GPI anchors.

2.1 N-glycans

This is the most prevalent and widely studied form of glycosylation. The glycan is bound via an N-glycosidic bond to an Asn residue within the consensus amino acid sequence (sequon) Asn-X-Ser/Thr. However, the presence of this sequon in a protein does not guarantee glycosylation. The glycosylation of the sequon is variable and gives rise to a macroheterogeneity of glycoforms (variable site occupancy). Amongst other factors, the site occupancy will depend upon the tertiary structure of the protein. There may be a multiplicity of glycan structures at a particular site. Differences in these structures is referred to as microheterogeneity.

The structures of N-linked glycans fall into three main categories: high-mannose, hybrid and complex type. They all have the same core structure, $Man_3GlcNAc_2$-Asn, but differ in their outer branches (*Figure 7.1*).

■ High-Mannose type: typically has two to six additional Man residues linked to the core.

■ Complex type: contains two or more outer branches containing N-acetyl glucosamine (GlcNAc), galactose (Gal), and sialic acid (SA).

■ Hybrid type: has features of both high-Man and complex type glycans.

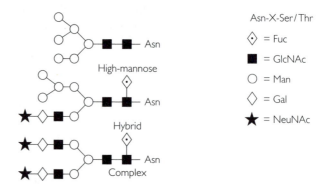

Figure 7.1

N-glycan structures of glycoproteins.

Common substituents to the N-glycan structures are Fucose (Fuc) linked to either the innermost core GlcNAc (proximal) or the outer arm GlcNAc (peripheral). Also, a 'bisecting' GlcNAc may be linked by β1,4 to the central core Man residue.

An alternative method of displaying these structures is shown in *Figure 7.2*. The advantage of this method is that the type of linkage between monosaccharides can be shown.

2.2   O-glycans

The glycan is bound via an O-glycosidic bond to a Ser/Thr (O-glycosylation). The most common are the O-linked mucin-type glycans, which are a heterogeneous group of structures. They can be classified into one of eight core structures that have been identified (*Figure 7.3*). Any Ser or Thr residue is a potential site for O-glycosylation and no consensus sequence in the protein has been identified.

2.3   GPI anchor

The glycan is a component of the glycosyl phosphatidylinositol (GPI) membrane anchor. This becomes an integral part of the cell membrane. This modification is absent in the secreted form of any glycoprotein and will not be considered further in this review.

3.   Assembly and processing of glycans on proteins

3.1   Assembly of N-linked glycans

This process is initiated in the endoplasmic reticulum as a protein is being synthesized from its constituent amino acids. The precursor glycan structure is added to the N-glycan sites and this is followed by a series of trimming reactions. High-mannose-type structures are formed during the processing in the ER. However, the completion of the processing to form hybrid and complex glycans takes place in the Golgi. A simplified version showing the formation of a complex biantennary structure is shown in *Figure 7.4*. The full diversity of glycan structures occurs because of a series of competing processing enzymes associated with this pathway.

All N-linked glycans on a glycoprotein share the same core because they all come from the same precursor which is transferred to the nascent protein

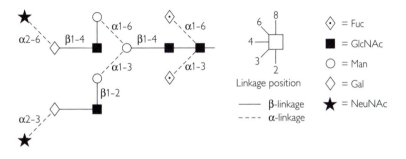

Figure 7.2

Di-sialylated biantennary structure showing linkage positions.

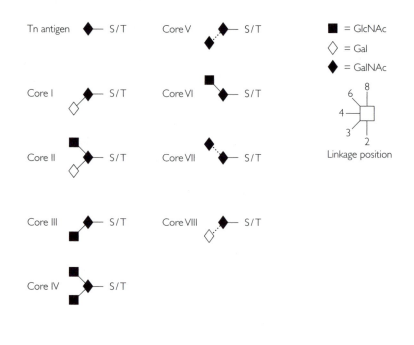

Figure 7.3

Core structures of mucin-type O-linked glycans.

in the endoplasmic reticulum. The precursor consists of a lipid (dolichol) linked to a glycan by a pyrophosphate bond. During synthesis of this glycan, sugars are added in a step-wise fashion, the first seven sugars (two GlcNAc and five Man) derive from the nucleotide sugars UDP-GlcNAc and GDP-Man respectively.

The next seven sugars (four Man and three Glc) are derived from the lipid intermediates Dol-P-Man and Dol-P-Glc. The final product, $Glc_3Man_9GlcNAc_2$-P-P-Dol, is the precursor for the N-linked glycans.

The glycosylation is initiated in the ER where the N-glycan precursor is attached to the consensus sequence Asn-X-Ser/Thr by the enzyme oligosaccharyltransferase. However, these sequences are not always glycosylated. Several factors can be identified that affect the attachment of a glycan to one of these sites.

- The spatial arrangements of the peptide during the translation process can expose or hide the tripeptide sequence.
- The amino acid sequence around the attachment site (Asn-X-Ser/Thr) is an important determinant of glycosylation efficiency. X can be any amino acid except Pro or Asp. The occupancy level is high when X= Ser, Phe, intermediate for Leu, Glu and very low for Asp, Trp and Pro.
- The availability of precursors (lipid, nucleotide sugars and correctly assembled precursor) level of expression of the oligosaccharyltransferase enzyme disulfide bond formation, which can make the site inaccessible to the precursor.

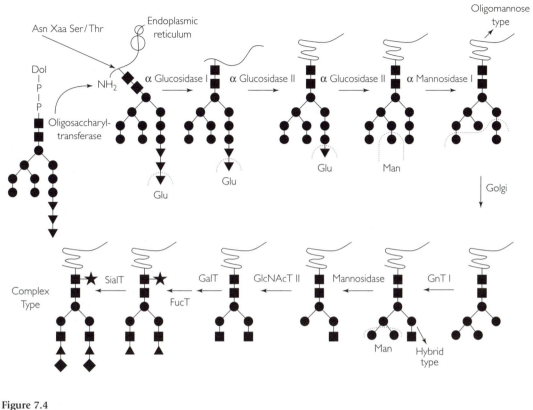

Figure 7.4

N-linked glycosylation pathway.

3.2 Glycan processing

Processing is initiated by a series of glucosidases, which are located in the membrane of the endoplasmic reticulum. The newly synthesized glycoproteins are then transported to the Golgi cisternae by means of vesicles.

In the Golgi a series of glycosidases and glycosyltransferases act on the N-linked glycans and lead to a diversity of structures (microheterogeneity). The final products can be modified further in the Golgi by the addition of:

- sialic acid: two main enzymes compete for the terminal Gal: $\alpha2,3$ sialyltransferase ($\alpha2,3$ST) and $\alpha2,6$ sialyltransferase ($\alpha2,6$ST);
- poly-N-acetyl lactosamine: it is added by βN-acetylglycosaminyltransferase (βGnT);
- fucose: by $\alpha1,6$ fucosyltransferase, that adds fucose in an $\alpha1,6$ linkage to the GlcNAc attached to Asn, or by $\alpha1,3$ fucosyltransferase that adds fucose to C3 of the GlcNAc residue in the sequence Gal $\beta1$–4 GlcNAc $\beta1$–2 Man. The product is not a substrate for the $\alpha2,6$ST. Fucose can be added at any time after M5 is synthesized but not after the action of Gal T or GnT III. Fucosylated glycans, however, can be modified by these enzymes.

The variety of glycans produced is a result of competitive activities of this range of enzymes. All the transferase-catalyzed reactions use sugar nucleotide co-substrates. It is evident that the key factor in determining the synthesis of particular N-linked glycans is the level of expression of the different glycosyltransferases.

The glycan profiles of glycoproteins are normally characteristic of the cell in which the protein is expressed and depends on cellular factors such as:

- enzyme repertoire;
- competition between different enzymes for one substrate;
- transit time of the glycoproteins;
- levels of sugar nucleotide donors;
- competition between different glycosylation sites on the protein for the same pool of enzymes.

At any time, many glycoproteins may be trafficking through the glycosylation pathway, competing for the glycosylation enzymes. The glycans attached to the glycoprotein are processed by some enzymes and not by others.

Umaña and Bailey (1997) proposed a mathematical model based on the activities of a set of eight enzymes and 32 reactions to determine the distribution of glycans into the major structural classes: high Man, hybrid, bisected hybrid, bi-, tri-, tri'- and tetraantennary complex and bisected complex glycans so the proportion of these structures could be calculated based on the kinetics of these enzymes.

3.3   Assembly of O-linked glycans

O-linked glycans are added post-translationally to the fully folded protein. Glycosylation can occur on exposed Ser or Thr residues but no consensus sequence has been identified.

The most commonly found O-glycans are the mucin-type, although other structures such as O-linked fucose or O-linked glucose do exist. The first step for the assembly of the mucin-type O-glycans is the addition of an N-acetylgalactosamine (GalNAc) residue to a Ser/Thr by a GalNAc transferase (GalNAcT) from UDP-GalNAc.

Although no consensus sequence has been identified for O-glycosylation, the glycosylated residue is often associated with regions of the peptide that contain a high proportion of Ser, Thr and Pro. It appears that this would make the polypeptide assume a favorable conformation making the Ser or Thr more accessible (Van den Steen *et al.*, 1998). Thr residues appear to be glycosylated more efficiently than Ser. Various GalNAcT have been identified, having a broad but different substrate specificity and are expressed in a tissue-specific manner. Further elongation leads to a large number of structures, synthesized by various glycosyltransferases, producing the eight different core structures (*Figure 7.3*). These core structures can be further modified by sialylation, fucosylation, sulfation, methylation or acetylation. A characteristic of transformed cells is that the initial GalNAc residue is not elongated and is known as the Tn antigen. Each of the core structures can give rise to a series of modified structures. An example of how metabolic engineering can lead to a modification of this metabolic network is discussed in Section 7.2.

4.   Glycoprotein analysis

Considerable advances have been made in the analysis of N-glycan structures over the last few years. These glycans can be separated from proteins by
a specific enzyme (N-PNGase F), a cleavage that can take place in isolated
bands from a protein gel (*Figure 7.5*). The isolated glycans may then be
labeled with a fluorescent dye and systematically degraded by specific exoglycosidases to give data related to the sequence of the glycan. Examples of

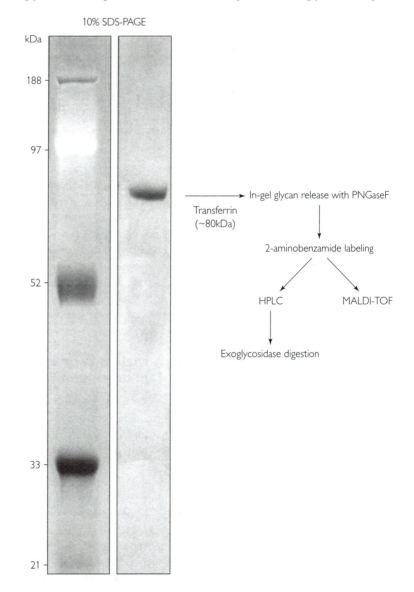

Figure 7.5

Glycoprotein analysis.

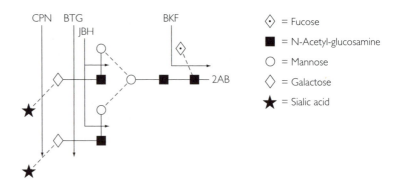

Figure 7.6

Specificity of exoglycosidase enzymes. Clostridium perfringens neuraminidase (CPN), Bovine testes β-galactosidase (BTG), Jack bean β-N-Acetylhexosaminidase (JBH). Bovine kidney α-fucosidase (BKF). Cleavage positions are shown by the arrows.

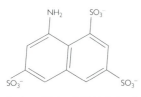

8-aminonaphthalene-1, 3, 6-trisulfonic acid

Figure 7.7

Fluorophore: ANTS.

these exoglycosidase enzymes are shown in *Figure 7.6*. Sequential addition of the enzymes results in a step-wise reduction in the size of the glycan and these products can be identified by HPLC. A suitable protocol is described at the end of this chapter (*Protocol 7.1*).

A simple method of glycan separation can also be provided by gel electrophoresis, providing the glycans are charged. The fluorophore, ANTS offers a suitable glycan label which provides both a negative charge and a fluorescent group for detection (*Figure 7.7*). A typical separation profile by fluorescence-activated carbohydrate electrophoresis (FACE) is shown in *Figure 7.8*.

5. Why mammalian cells are chosen for glycoprotein production

The prokaryotes (mainly *E. coli*) were the first cells to be used for gene expression of recombinant proteins. These cells can be easily manipulated and grown in large scale but they lack the necessary glycosylation machinery and so the proteins produced are not glycosylated.

An alternative is offered by lower eukaryotes (yeast, insect and plant cells). However, the glycans produced in these cells differ significantly from those present in human glycoproteins. Yeast, insect, plant and mammalian cells share the feature of N-linked glycan processing in the endoplasmic reticulum, including attachment of $Glc_3Man_9GlcNAc_2$-P-P-Dol and subsequent truncation to $Man_8GlcNAc_2$ structure. However, glycan processing by these different cell types diverges in the Golgi apparatus. Although there is extensive heterogeneity of structures arising from any cell type, examples of predominant N-glycans that might occur from different systems are shown in *Table 7.1*.

Mammalian cells are the chosen host for the production of human glycoproteins because it has been recognized that they meet the criteria for an appropriate glycosylation of recombinant human glycoproteins. They are capable of complex-type N-glycan processing whereas the other systems are

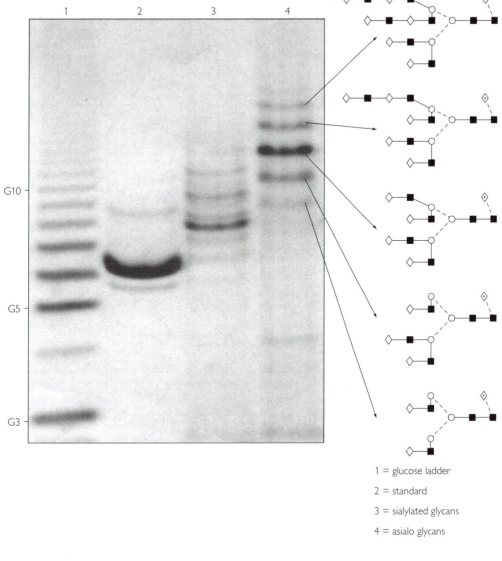

1 = glucose ladder

2 = standard

3 = sialylated glycans

4 = asialo glycans

Figure 7.8

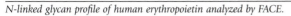

N-linked glycan profile of human erythropoietin analyzed by FACE.

not. However, there are different capabilities for glycosylation between mammalian cell lines as discussed in Section 6.1. The most commonly used cell lines for recombinant protein production are the hamster-derived Chinese hamster ovary (CHO) and baby hamster kidney (BHK) cells. These cell lines have been chosen because of their favorable growth characteristics in culture as anchorage-dependent or suspension cells. They have been used as expression systems to produce proteins whose glycoforms are similar to the native human products.

Table 7.1. Typical predominant N-glycan structures from different cell types

Cell type	N-glycan	Structure
Bacteria, *E. coli*	None	-------------
Yeast	High mannose	
Insect	Fucosylated core structure	
Plant	Xylosylated and fucosylated core structure	
Mammalian	Complex biantennary	

Symbols: N-acetyl glucosamine (■); mannose (○), fucose (◇), xylose (△), galactose (◇), sialic acid (★)

6. Control of glycan processing in mammalian cell culture

6.1 Host cell

The glycan structures on the same proteins can vary between species and even different tissues. The level of expression of the various glycosyltransferases is a key factor in the synthesis of the N-linked glycans. Differences in the relative activity of these enzymes among species and tissues can account for many of the variations in glycan structures that are present.

An analysis of the glycan structures of IgG from 13 different species shows that there is significant variation in the proportion of terminal galactose, core fucose and bisecting GlcNAc. The predominant monosaccharide precursors may also differ structurally between species. For example the terminal sialic acid found in glycoproteins from goats, sheep and cows is predominantly N-glycolyl-neuraminic acid (NGNA) rather than N-acetyl-neuraminic acid (NANA) which is the sialic acid structure generally found in humans and rodents.

CHO and BHK are the most commonly used cell lines for the production of recombinant proteins with potential application as therapeutic agents. For such an application it would be desirable to obtain proteins with as near a human glycosylation profile as possible. However both CHO and BHK show differences in their potential for glycosylation compared to human cells. The sialyltransferase enzyme, α2,6ST is not active in these cell lines, leading to exclusively α2,3-linked terminal SA residues. Furthermore, the absence of a functional α1,3 fucosyltransferase in CHO cells prevents the addition of peripheral Fuc residues and also the absence of N-acetylglu-cosaminyltransferase III (GnT III) prevents the addition of bisecting GlcNAc.

However, the differences in glycosylation capabilities between CHO and human cells do not appear to result in glycoproteins that are immunogenic. Natural human erythropoietin (EPO) consists of a mixture of sialylated forms – 60% being 2,3-linked and 40% being 2,6-linked. Because of the restricted sialylation capacity of CHO cells, the recombinant EPO is sialyl-ated entirely via the α2,3 linkages. Nevertheless, recombinant EPO produced from CHO cells is currently employed as a highly effective therapeutic agent in the treatment of a variety of renal dysfunctions. There is no evidence of any adverse physiological effect due to the structural difference in the terminal sialic acid.

Mouse cells express the enzyme α1,3 galactosyltransferase, which gener-ates Galα1,3-Galβ1,4-GlcNAc residues not present in humans and is an epitope found to be highly immunogenic. The epitope is found in the glycan structures of glycoproteins from nonprimate animals including rodents, pigs, sheep and cows as well as New World monkeys. Although there is evi-dence for the presence of the gene of this enzyme in CHO and BHK cells, there appears to be no activity of the α1,3 galactosyltransferase enzyme. The potential for immunogenicity associated with this epitope limits the use of murine cells for therapeutic glycoprotein production. Some of the charac-teristics of the glycosylation capacity of CHO cells and murine C127 cells are summarized in *Table 7.2*.

Genetic mutations can also affect glycan synthesis. A series of CHO clones has been isolated possessing a variety of mutations affecting N- and O-glycosylation. The mutants are characterized by the expression of aberrant lectins on the cell surface and are classified as a series of numbered LEC mutants. These mutations usually diminish the glycosylation capability. For example, Lec1 CHO mutant expresses no detectable GnT I and accumulates glycoproteins with $Man_5GlcNAc_2$ structures in the cell. A mutant affected in the same gene, Lec1A was isolated from a sub-population of this mutant. This mutant produces a GnT I biochemically different from the one produced by the parental cell line, with new kinetic properties (Chaney and Stanley,

Table 7.2. Characteristics of the glycosylation capacity of two widely used mammalian cell lines compared to normal human cells

I. CHO cells

- lacks α2,6 sialyltransferase activity. Sialylation by CHO cells only produces α2,3 linkages to terminal N-glycan structures
- unable to sulfate GalNAc residues. This is important in certain hormones
- lacks α1,3 fucosyltransferase. This prevents the formation of peripheral fucose residues (Fuc-α1,3-GlcNAc)
- lacks β1,4 N-acetylglucosaminyltransferase III. This prevents the formation of GlcNAc attachment to the core mannose to form a bisected glycan

2. Murine C127 cells

- lacks α2,3 sialyltransferase activity. Sialylation by C127 cells only produces α2,6 linkages to terminal N-glycan structures
- expresses α1,3 galactosyltransferase activity. This results in Gal-α1,3-Gal which is antigenic in humans

1986). Multiple enzymic defects may be an advantage in the production of glycoproteins with minimal carbohydrate heterogeneity (Stanley, 1989).

A mutation may also result in a mutant with a gain of function such as the CHO Lec11, which expresses α1,3 fucosyltransferase. CHO cells have a limited capacity for synthesis of elongated O-glycans because of the lack of core 2 GlcNAcT activity, although this enzyme may be induced by butyrate treatment.

6.2   Culture environment

The control of the culture environment is important to maximize cell growth in order to attain a high cell density, which is a prerequisite for producing cell products whether they be viruses, antibodies or recombinant proteins. However, it is also important to realize that the specific conditions of the culture can affect product glycosylation independently of the characteristics of the cell line. During the course of a batch culture nutrient consumption and product accumulation change the cellular environment, usually in a way that can gradually decrease the extent of protein glycosylation over time. Such changes are unacceptable in a cell culture bioprocess used for large-scale production of a protein that may be a therapeutic agent. It can lead to variable glycoform heterogeneity and significant batch-to-batch variation in the production processes. In order to maintain product consistency it is essential to understand the parameters of cell culture that can cause variations in glycosylation. As a more far-reaching objective it may be reasonable to control culture conditions in favor of reducing glycoform heterogeneity or producing a specific glycoform. For example, the maximization of product sialylation of therapeutic proteins could lead to higher specific biological activities *in vivo*.

Two lines of evidence suggest that the extracellular environment may affect glycosylation: (a) *in vivo* changes in glycosylation are associated with the physiological state, e.g. pregnancy and disease (e.g. diabetes); (b) *in vitro* cell culture studies show direct effects of the extracellular environment on protein glycosylation. In some cases these have been reported from changes in the mode of culture. For example, the glycosylation of antibodies was found to be more consistent by *in vitro* culture than from ascites fluid or from the adaptation of cells from serum to serum-free medium. In other reports, the specific culture parameters affecting an alteration in glycosylation have been analyzed.

The choice of culture method, pH, nutrient concentration, dissolved oxygen, etc., are some of the parameters that may affect the glycan structures of glycoproteins. Among the potential mechanisms to explain such effects are:

- depletion of the cellular energy state;
- disruption of the local ER and Golgi environment;
- modulation of glycosidase and glycosyltransferase activities;
- modulation of the synthesis of nucleotides, nucleotide sugars and lipid precursors.

The awareness of such effects on the glycosylation of proteins makes the use of more defined culture media and conditions a very important issue for the development of a pharmaceutical product with defined glycan structures and batch consistency.

6.3   Mode of culture

CHO and BHK cells can be grown as anchorage-dependent cells in T-flasks or microcarriers. Alternatively, they can be adapted to suspension culture. This adaptation process leads to characteristic changes in the expression of cell surface proteins such as the integrins which affect viral susceptibility. Not surprisingly, the glycosylation process may also be affected by such changes. Watson *et al.* (1994) reported that the sialylation of N-glycans of a secreted protein from CHO was reduced in microcarrier culture compared to suspension. Gawlitzek *et al.* (1995) also showed an effect on glycan antennarity of a BHK-produced protein related to the mode of culture.

The presence or absence of serum in the culture medium also has a significant effect on glycosylation. This is not surprising given the variable concentrations of hormones and growth factors in serum and even in different formulations of serum-free media. Cells grown in SFM (serum-free medium) secrete a higher proportion of N-glycosylated and O-glycosylated protein with enhanced terminal sialylation and proximal fucosylation. This result was attributed to the presence of high activities of sialidase and fucosidase in serum.

6.4   Protein productivity

Differences in growth rate, specific productivity and cell density among the bioreactors may cause variations in the pattern of N-linked glycan structures, especially in the degree of sialylation. This has been shown in experiments using different bioreactors established under similar conditions (Schweikart *et al.*, 1999). It has also been shown that the rate of protein expression may affect glycosylation. In one set of experiments the slower transit time of the glycoproteins through the Golgi at lower temperatures was shown to increase the number of polylactosamine residues in the glycans (Nabi and Dennis, 1998).

6.5   Glucose

Low glucose concentrations may produce two distinct abnormalities in the synthesis of glycoproteins: attachment of aberrant precursors to the protein and absence of glycosylation at sites that are normally glycosylated. Both abnormalities are due to a shortage of glucose-derived glycan precursors. Glucose starvation may result in an intracellular energy-depleted state or a shortage of glucose-derived glycan precursors. Reduced site occupancy of Ig light chains was observed in mouse myeloma cells grown at a glucose concentration below 0.5 mM. Abnormal glycosylation of viral proteins is also observed at low glucose. In a chemostat culture of CHO cells Hayter *et al.* (1993) showed an increase in nonglycosylated gamma-interferon under glucose-limiting conditions. Pulsed additions of glucose restored normal glycosylation rapidly.

6.6   Ammonia

Glutamine is normally added to culture medium at a concentration of 2–10 mM. The glutamine provides an energy source for cells as well as being an essential precursor for nucleotide synthesis. However, glutamine is a source of ammonia accumulation in culture medium which arises from either thermal decomposition of the glutamine or from metabolic deamination or deamidation. The accumulated ammonia is inhibitory to cell growth and also has a specific effect on protein glycosylation. Ammonia is likely to cause a decrease in sialylation and a change in the number of antennae of the glycan.

There are two major changes to the intracellular environment caused by ammonia that could explain its effect on glycosylation.

■   An increase in pH of the Golgi. This could decrease the activity of selected enzymes.
■   An increase in the UDP-GNAc pool. This could compete with the transport of CMP-NeuAc into the Golgi that is necessary for sialylation.

6.7   pH

Under adverse external pH conditions the internal pH of the Golgi is likely to change, resulting in a reduction of the activities of key glycosylating enzymes. The pH of the medium has been shown to affect the distribution of glycoforms of IgG secreted by a murine hybridoma. It has also been shown that the maximum glycan occupancy of a protein occurs between pH values of 6.9 and 8.2 (Borys et al., 1993).

6.8   Dissolved oxygen concentration

Oxygen plays a dominant role in the metabolism and viability of cells; it is a limiting nutrient in animal cell culture because of its low solubility in the medium. It has also been shown to affect the pattern of glycans on a protein expressed by cells in culture. Monoclonal antibodies have a biantennary glycan structure at a site on the heavy chains that may show two (G2), one (G1) or no (G0) terminal galactose groups. A decrease in galactosylation may occur at reduced dissolved oxygen (DO) concentrations (10% DO), when mainly agalactosyl or monogalactosylated glycans occur while at higher oxygen concentration (50–100% DO) there is a higher proportion of digalactosylated glycans (Figure 15 in Kunkel et al., 1998).

The mechanism for the effect of DO on galactosylation is unclear. One explanation is that reduced DO causes a decline in the availability of the UDP-Gal. This might arise due to a sensitivity to reduced oxidative phosphorylation in the production of UDP-Gal or as a result of reduced UDP-Gal transport from the cytosol to the Golgi. A second explanation is based on evidence that the timing and rate of formation of the inter-heavy chain disulfide bonds in the hinge region of IgG determine the level of Fc galactosylation (Rademacher et al., 1996). Thus the addition of galactose may be impeded by the early formation of the inter-heavy chain disulfide bond. Low DO in the culture may cause a perturbation in the oxidating environment of the ER and/or the Golgi complex and the disturbance may result in a change in the pathway of inter-chain disulfide bond formation.

An effect of DO has also been observed in CHO cultures, with enhanced sialylation of a recombinant protein at high oxygen levels (Chotigeat et al., 1994).

6.9   Growth factors/cytokines/hormones

There are many reports of hormones involved in the regulation of protein glycosylation in vivo. Up- and down-regulation of specific glycosyltransferases has been observed frequently in conjunction with hormonal induction of cell differentiation. Presumably, transcriptional control of glycosylation enzyme concentration is responsible for many of the effects on glycan processing. An example of glycosylation control *in vivo* is the cascade of events that occurs following the stimulation of the synthesis of thyrotropin by the tripeptide, thyrotropin-releasing hormone (TRH). This in turn promotes the synthesis and sialylation of thyroglobulin by thyroid cells. The glycosylation of transferrin is regulated by prolactin in rabbit mammary glands.

In cell culture dexamethasone can affect glycan structures in rat hepatocytes. Retinol and retinoic acid may play a role *in vivo* in epithelial cell differentiation and can be shown in culture to cause significant changes to protein glycosylation. This includes a shift from high mannose to complex glycans in chondrocytes and the extension of complex structures in mouse melanoma cells.

Exogenous IL-6 induces changes in the activities of intracellular GnTs including a reduction in the activity of GnT III and an increase in GnT IV and GnT V of a myeloma cell line that led to alterations in the glycan structure of the surface and secreted glycoproteins (Nakas *et al.*, 1990).

6.10 Extracellular degradation of glycans

Mammalian cells possess glycosidases that may be released extracellularly into the culture by cell secretion or upon cell lysis. These include fucosidases, β galactosidases, β hexosaminidases and sialidases that may accumulate in the extracellular medium. CHO cells possess a significant and stable sialidase activity that can accumulate in the culture medium and retains considerable activity at pH 7 (Gramer and Goochee, 1993). The action of these enzymes on secreted glycoproteins that have a variable residence time in the culture may result in significant heterogeneity of glycoforms.

The extent of glycan degradation depends on many factors, including the level of extracellular activity, pH, temperature and time of the glycoprotein exposure to the enzyme. Bioprocesses that result in maintenance of high cell densities for long periods such as fed-batch or perfusion mode cultures may be particularly vulnerable to this type of glycan degradation. Early extraction of the product from the medium reduces the residence time of the glycoprotein in culture and may reduce glycoform heterogeneity.

7. Genetic engineering of mammalian cells to modify glycosylation

Mammalian cell lines used for the production of glycoproteins may lack the enzymic profile to synthesize recombinant proteins that are glycosylated as authentic human proteins. This may be due to the lack of processing enzymes, the presence of alternative processing enzymes or through the expression of glycosidase activities in the mammalian host cells.

Metabolic engineering provides a promising tool to modify the characteristics of the host mammalian cells by enhancing cell productivity, protein quality and bioactivity and by modifying the glycosylation pathway to obtain a final product with advantageous properties.

7.1   Engineering host cells for new glycosylation properties

The two commonly used hamster cell lines, BHK-21 and CHO cells do not express α2,6 sialyltransferase, α1,3 fucosyltransferase or β-1,4-N-acetylglucosaminyltransferase III activities. As these enzymes are found in normal human cells, the products of the hamster cell lines may not possess some of the glycan structures found typically in human serum proteins.

Transfection of the cells with the gene of the lacking glycosyltransferase may correct such deficiencies.

α2,6 Sialyltransferase (α2,6ST)

Two different sialic acid linkages (α2,3 and α2,6) to the terminal Gal are found in N-linked glycans isolated from human glycoproteins. The human enzymes responsible for these substitutions are α2,3ST and α2,6ST. Both enzymes compete for the same substrate and a mixture of both linkages is often found in native human glycoproteins. However, CHO and BHK-21 cells only produce α2,3 sialylated glycan structures.

The sialyltransferase (α2,6ST) gene has been introduced into BHK cells that express recombinant proteins (Grabenhorst et al., 1995). The modified cells produced glycoproteins with an increased level of sialylation which included a mixture of 2,3/6 sialylated glycan structures.

Similarly, CHO cells have been co-transfected with genes for IFN-γ and α2,6ST (Lamotte et al., 1999). The modified cells produced IFN-γ, 68% of which was sialylated with a α2,6 linkage. The overall extent of sialylation was doubled compared to the product of the cells without the α2,6ST gene. The addition of sodium butyrate enhanced the α2,6ST activity and increased the extent of sialylation and the proportion of α2,6 linked SA to 82%. However, sodium butyrate had no effect on the sialylation of the product of the cells without the α2,6ST gene insert.

α1,3 Fucosyltransferase (α1,3FT)

This enzyme is required for the addition of a peripheral α1,3 fucose linkage to GlcNAc as found in certain human proteins. The co-expression of β-TP from recombinant BHK-21 cells with human α1,3FT successfully produced a glycoprotein, 50% of which had an α1,3-linked Fuc (Grabenhorst et al., 1999). However, a significant decrease in the degree of sialylation of N-glycans was observed. It is suggested that this could be due to competition of α1,3FT with the endogenous α2,3ST for the same substrate. The α2,3 sialyltransferase is unable to sialylate fucosylated structures.

β1,4 N-acetyl glucosaminyltransferase (GnT III)

The bisecting GlcNAc residue plays an important role in the branching and elongation of glycan structures by restricting the action of other enzymes. GnT III is not expressed at significant levels in normal CHO cells so the synthesis of bisected glycans does not occur in these cells unless they are transferred with the GnT III gene.

A CHO cell line capable of producing bisected glycans on the glycan structure of IFN-β has been created (Sburlati et al., 1998). This structure has not been detected in native human IFN-β and the biological significance of this is unknown.

Immunoglobulin glycosylation is essential for complement fixation and antibody-dependent mediated cytotoxicity (ADCC). This is a lytic attack on antibody-targeted cells and is initiated after the binding of a lymphocyte receptor to the constant region (Fc) of the antibodies. This effector function may be essential for the therapeutic application of certain antibodies. Although human serum IgG contains low levels of bisecting GlcNAc, therapeutic antibodies containing bisected glycans may have an enhanced ADCC.

One example of this is a chimeric IgG1 (chCE7) anti-neuroblastoma engineered in CHO cells which showed enhanced ADCC as a result of the presence of bisected glycoforms in the Fc region (Umana et al., 1999). The antibody chCE7 was constructed by transfecting the CHO parental cell line with the GnT III gene under tetracycline regulation. Over-expression of GnT III led to a modified IgG containing a bisected glycoform. The maximal activity of ADCC correlated with a high level of Fc-associated bisected complex glycans. Thus, enhanced ADCC activity of chCE7 together with the capacity of this antibody to recognize neuroblastoma cells, makes it a suitable candidate molecule for the treatment of these tumors.

The effect of GnT III expression levels on glycan structures in CHO cells was predicted by a mathematical model based upon enzyme kinetic constants and mass balances associated with the production of 33 different N-glycan structures (Umana and Bailey, 1997). GnT III has the potential to act upon at least seven independent glycan structures that result in either bisected complex and bisected hybrid glycans. The complex form is the required structure to maximize biological activity *in vivo*. Analysis of the competitive enzymic reactions in the central reaction network of the Golgi can be used to predict the activity of GnT III required to maximize synthesis of the bisected complex glycoforms.

7.2 Metabolic regulation of O-glycosylation

The predominant O-glycan structures formed in CHO cells are the core I type (*Figure 7.3*). However it has been shown by the simultaneous up-regulation and down-regulation of key enzymes that this pathway can be altered. CHO cells that had been genetically engineered to express α1,3 fucosyltransferase (α1,3FT) were selected for the co-expression of a CMP-sialic acid: Galβ1,3GalNAcα2,3-sialyltransferase (ST3Gal I) gene fragment set in the antisense orientation and the human UDP-GlcNAc:Galβ1,3GalNAc-R β1,6-N-acetylglucosaminyltransferase (C2GnT) (Prati et al., 2000). This co-expression resulted in an increase in the activity of the C2GnT enzyme and a decrease in the activity of the ST3Gal I enzyme. The effect of this coordinated change was to divert the O-glycosylation pathway from the formation of core I glycans to core II glycans. The significance of this is the formation of proteins containing sialyl-Lewis X glycan structures that mediate interaction with selectins and cell–cell adhesion.

7.3 Antisense RNA and gene targeting for altered glycosylation

An alternative for metabolic engineering of producer mammalian cells focuses on the direct manipulation of the expression of endogenous proteins by the use of antisense RNA. This approach is suitable for removing an unwanted enzyme activity or to enhance the expression of endogenous proteins to improve the product quality or enhance cell productivity.

One obvious target for this strategy in CHO cells is the soluble sialidase gene. A reduction of sialidase expression would improve the stability of secreted proteins in culture supernatant. The de-sialylation of therapeutic proteins reduces bioactivity because the resulting proteins with exposed terminal Gal residues are removed from the bloodstream by hepatocyte asialo-glycoprotein receptors. Thus, the conservation of sialic acid in the glycan chains of glycoproteins is critical and must be maintained on the proteins during the production and purification processes.

Antisense expression of sialidase resulted in a 60% reduction of sialidase activity in the culture supernatant of CHO cells expressing DNAase (Ferrari *et al.*, 1998). Although only an additional one mole of sialic acid per mole of protein was observed, this modest improvement in sialylation resulted in a dramatic effect on the serum clearance rate of the protein.

Antisense RNA targeting has proven to be a valuable means to revive silent genes or correct gene defects. More complete glycosylation of recombinant glycoproteins may be possible if the activities of endogenous glycosyltransferases are increased above normal levels (Warner, 1999).

Two strategies for the construction of antisense expressing cells are possible: (i) The creation of a universal host cell line which expresses the desired antisense RNA. Once the cell line is established, the product expression vector is introduced. The advantage of this approach is the availability of a universal cell line constitutively expressing antisense RNA. (ii) The introduction of the antisense expression vector into an existing recombinant host after growth and productivity parameters have been optimized. This reduces the possibility of modifying the antisense RNA.

8.   Conclusion

The choice of the cell expression systems and the control of the production parameters at earlier stages of bioprocess development are key factors for ensuring the production of glycoproteins with consistent structures.

To optimize the glycoform distribution for a given glycoprotein produced by a given cell type it is important to understand the specific environmental factors affecting glycan structures and how to control these factors at the cellular level. Given the biological complexities of cell growth and metabolism, the cellular and environmental parameters that can be potentially altered are enormous. An increased awareness of the importance of pharmaceutical protein glycosylation has led to the increased importance of analysis of glycan structures.

Recent efforts in metabolic engineering are clearly justified in view of the demands for the production of proteins with a consistent glycoform profile and more cost-effective, high-productivity processes. Continuing efforts in metabolic engineering may lead to host cell lines capable of producing a restricted set of glycoforms for a specific glycoprotein, with enhanced bioactivity and reduced blood clearance rates.

References

Borys, M.C., Linzer, D.I.H. and Papoutsakis, E.T. (1993) Culture pH affects expression rates and glycosylation of recombinant mouse placental lactogen proteins by Chinese hamster ovary (CHO) cells. *Biotechnology* 11: 720–724.

Chaney, W. and Stanley, P. (1986) Lec1A Chinese hamster ovary cell mutants appear to arise from a structural alteration in N-acetylglycosaminyltransferase I. *J. Biochem. Chem.* **261**: 10551–10557.

Chotigeat, W., Watanapokasin, Y., Mahler, S., and Gray, P.P. (1994) Role of environmental conditions on the expression levels, glycoform pattern and levels of sialyltransferase for hFSH produced by recombinant CHO cells. *Cytotechnology* **15**: 217–221.

Ferrari J., Gunson J., Lofgren J., Krummen L. and Warner T.G. (1998) Chinese hamster ovary cells with constitutively expressed sialidase antisense RNA produce recombinant DNase in batch culture with increased sialic acid. *Biotech. Bioeng.* **60**: 589–595.

Gawlitzek, M., Valley, U., Nimtz, M., Wagner, R. and Conradt, H.S. (1995) Characterization of changes in the glycosylation pattern of recombinant proteins from BHK-21 cells due to different culture conditions. *J. Biotech.* **42**: 117–131.

Grabenhorst, E., Hoffmann, A., Nimtz, M., Zettlmeissl, G. and Conradt, H.S. (1995) Construction of stable BHK-21 cells coexpressing human secretory glycoprotein and human Gal (β1–4)GlcNAc-R α2,6-sialyltransferase. *Eur. J. Biochem.* **232**: 718–725.

Grabenhorst, E., Schlenke, P., Pohl, S., Nimtz, M. and Conradt, H.S. (1999) Genetic engineering of recombinant glycoproteins and the glycosylation pathway in mammalian host cells. *Glycoconjugate J.* **16**: 81–97.

Gramer, M.J. and Goochee, C.F. (1993) Glycosidase activities in Chinese hamster ovary cell lysate and cell culture supernatant. *Biotechnol. Prog.* **9**: 366–373.

Guile, G.R., Rudd, P.M., Wing, D.R., Prime, S.B. and Dwek, R.A. (1996) A rapid high-resolution high-performance liquid chromatographic method for separating glycan mixtures and analyzing oligosaccharide profiles. *Anal Biochem.* **240**: 210–226.

Hayter, P.M., Curling, E.M., Gould, M.L., Baines, A.J., Jenkins, N., Salmon, I., Strange, P.G. and Bull, A.T. (1993) The effect of dilution rate on CHO cell physiology and recombinant interferon γ production in glucose-limited chemostat cultures. *Biotech. Bioeng* **42**: 1077–1085.

Jenkins, N. and Curling, E.M. (1994) Glycosylation of recombinant proteins: problems and prospects. *Enzyme Microbial Technol.* **16**: 354–364.

Jenkins, N., Parekh, R.B. and James, D.C. (1996) Getting the glycosylation right: Implications for the biotechnology industry. *Nat. Biotechnol.* **14**: 975–981.

Kunkel, J.P., Jan, D.C.H., Jamieson, J.C. and Butler, M. (1998) Dissolved oxygen concentration in serum-free continuous culture affects N-linked glycosylation of a monoclonal antibody. *J. Biotechnol.* **62**: 55–71.

Lamotte, D., Buckberry, L., Monaco, L., Soria, M., Jenkins, N., Engasser, J-M. and Marc A. (1999) Na-butyrate increases the production and α2,6-sialylation of recombinant interferon-γ expressed by α2,6-sialyltransferase engineered CHO cells. *Cytotechnology* **29**: 55–64.

Nabi, I.R. and Dennis, J.W. (1998) The extent of polylactosamine glycosylation of MDCK LAMP-2 is determined by its Golgi residence time. *Glycobiology* **8**: 947–953.

Nakao, H., Nishikawa, A., Karasuno, T., Nishiura, T., Iida, M., Kanayama, Y., Yonezawa, T., Tarui, S. and Taniguchi, N. (1990) Modulation of N-acetylglucosaminyltransferase III, IV and V activities and alteration of the surface oligosaccharide structure of a myeloma cell line by interleukin 6. *Biochem. Biophys Res Commun.* **172**: 1260–1266.

Prati, E.G.P., Matasci, M., Suter, T.B., Dinter, A., Sburlati, A.R., and Bailey, J.E. (2000) Engineering of co-ordinated up- and down-regulation of two glycotransferases of the o-glycosylation pathway in Chinese hamster ovary (CHO) cells. *Biotechnol. Bioeng.* **68**: 239–244.

Rademacher, T.W., Jaques, A. and Williams, P.J. (1996) The defining characteristics of immunoglobulin glycosylation. In: Isenberg, D.A. and Rademacher, T.W. (eds) *Abnormalities of IgG Glycosylation and Immunological Disorders*, pp. 1–44. Wiley, New York.

Rudd, P.M. and Dwek, R.A. (1997) Glycosylation: Heterogeneity and the 3D structure of proteins. *Crit. Rev. Biochem. Molec. Biol.* **32**: 1–100.

Sburlati, A.R., Umaña, P., Prati, E.G. and Bailey, J.E. (1998) Synthesis of bisected glycoforms of recombinant IFN-β by over expression of β-1,4-N-acetyl glucosaminyltransferase III in Chinese hamster ovary cells. *Biotechnol. Prog.* **14**: 189–192.

Schweikart, F., Jones, R., Jaton, J.C. and Hughes, G.J. (1999) Rapid structural characterization of a murine monoclonal IgA α-chain: heterogeneity in the oligosaccharide structures at a specific site in samples produced in different bioreactor systems. *J. Biotechnol.* **69**: 191–201.

Stanley, P. (1989) Chinese hamster ovary cell mutants with multiple glycosylation defects for production of glycoproteins with minimal carbohydrate heterogeneity. *Mol. Cell. Biol.* **9**: 377–383.

Umaña, P. and Bailey, J.E. (1997) A mathematical model of N-linked glycoform biosynthesis. *Biotechnol. Bioeng.* **55**: 890–908.

Umaña, P., Jean-Mairet, J., Moudry, R., Amstuz, H. and Bailey, J.E. (1999). Engineered glycoforms of an antineuroblastoma IgG1 optimized antibody-dependent cellular cytotoxic activity. *Nature Biotech.* **17**: 176–180.

Van den Steen, P., Rudd, P.M., Dwek, R.A. and Opdenakker, G. (1998) Concepts and principles of O-linked glycosylation. *Crit. Rev. Biochem. Mol. Biol.* **33**: 151–208.

Warner T.G. (1999) Enhancing therapeutic glycoprotein production in Chinese hamster ovary cells by metabolic engineering endogenous gene control with anti-sense DNA and gene targeting. *Glycobiology* **9**: 841–850.

Watson, E., Shah, B., Leiderman, L., Hsu, Y.R., Karkare, S., Lu, H.S. and Lin, F.K. (1994) Comparison of N-linked oligosaccharides of recombinant human tissue kallikrein produced from Chinese hamster ovary cells on microcarrier beads and in serum-free suspension culture. *Biotechnol. Prog.* **10**: 39–44.

Further reading

Al-Rubeai, M. (2002) *Cell Engineering: Glycosylation*. Kluwer, Dordrecht.

Brooks, S.A., Dwek, M.V. and Schumacher, U. (2002) *Functional and Molecular Glycobiology*. BIOS Scientific, Oxford.

Fukuda, M. and Hindsgaul, O. (2000) *Molecular and Cellular Glycobiology (Frontiers in Molecular Biology, 30)*. Oxford University Press, Oxford.

Fukuda, M. and Kobata, A. (1997) *Glycobiology: A Practical Approach*. IRL Press, Oxford.

Lennarz, W.J., Hart, G.W. and Simon, M.J. (1994) *Guide to Techniques in Glycobiology*. Academic Press, San Diego.

Taylor, M.E. and Drickamer, K. (2002) *Introduction to Glycobiology*. Oxford University Press, Oxford.

Townsend, R.R. and Hotchkiss, A.T. Jr. (1997) *Techniques in Glycobiology*. Marcel Dekker, New York.

Varki, A., Cummings, R., Esko, J. *et al.* (1999) *The Essentials of Glycobiology*. Cold Spring Harbor, New York.

Protocol 7.1

Analysis of glycans from in-gel release of protein bands

Materials

0.5 M dithiothreitol (DTT)

100 mM iodoacetamide (IAA)

NuPage 10% gel with MOPS pH 7 as running buffer

Sodium bicarbonate buffer 20 mM, pH 7

PNGase F (Boehringer) 1 unit/ml

Dowex AG50 X12 anion exchange resin

GlycoClean S cartridge (Glyko)

2-aminobenzamide (2-AB) labeling reagent (Glyko)

Procedure

1. Reduce a protein sample (50–70 μg) with DTT for 10 min.

2. Alkylate sample with iodoacetamide for 30 min.

3. Apply protein samples (5–10 μg) to individual gel lanes for separation by SDS-PAGE with precast gels and MOPS running buffer.

4. Stain gel with Coomassie Blue to reveal distinct protein bands.

5. Remove the protein bands from three identical lanes from the stained gel by scalpel. Cut into small pieces (1 mm^2) and transfer to an Eppendorf tube.

6. Freeze the tube for at least 2 h to break up gel prior to enzymic digestion.

7. Wash alternately with sodium bicarbonate buffer 20 mM, pH 7 and aceto-nitrile.

8. Treat the dried gel pieces with PNGase F enzyme (3 μl) and sodium bicarbonate buffer (27 μl) for 12–16 h at 37°C to remove the attached glycans.

9. Extract the glycans from the gel pieces by repeated (×3) sonication with 200 μl water for 30 min.

10. De-salt the extract by passage through a 0.5 ml Dowex AG50 X12 column and elution with 4 × 0.5 ml water. Dry the sample completely prior to labeling.

11. Label each sample by reductive amination with the fluorophore, 2-amino-benzamide (5 μl) at 5°C for 2 h.

12. Remove excess labeling reagent by acetonitrile elution through a GlycoClean S cartridge. The sample elutes subsequently with water. Alternatively, ascending paper chromatography (Whatman 3 MM filter paper) with acetonitrile can remove the reagent.

13. Each labeled glycan sample can be analyzed by normal phase HPLC.

14. Structural assignment of the peaks arising from this separation can be performed by subsequent treatment with multi-enzyme arrays of exoglycosidases (Guille et al., 1996).

Chapter 8

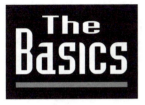

Hybridomas – sources of antibodies

1. Introduction

Since the 1970s, monoclonal antibodies have become essential tools for most research laboratories involved in cell and molecular biology. They have also been used to develop routine diagnostic medical tests and more recently as therapeutic agents.

The purpose of this chapter is to describe the background to the methods used to produce hybridomas that secrete monoclonal antibodies (Mabs) and to show how this can be done in the laboratory. The techniques described can be performed in any cell culture laboratory with access to animal facilities. Alternatively, a wide range of antibody-secreting hybridomas is available from culture collections.

2. Antibody production *in vivo*

Antibodies are found in a specific protein fraction of blood called the gamma-globulin or the immunoglobulin fraction. They are synthesized by a subset of white blood cells – the B-lymphocytes. The basic structural arrangement of two heavy associated with two light chains is similar for all the isotypes. However, each isotype is distinguished by different heavy chain structures, which are of varying length, number of domains and glycan structures.

Each B-lymphocyte is capable of producing one type of antibody in response to a particular antigen which interacts with a cell surface receptor. Stimulation by an antigen causes growth and an expansion of the cell population capable of producing the corresponding antibody. The variety of antibodies present in any animal reflects the population of B-lymphocytes which have been stimulated by previous exposure to a range of antigens.

A particular antibody will be produced in an animal following the injection of the corresponding antigen. For example, if human insulin is injected into a mouse, after a few days the blood will contain significant quantities of mouse antibody capable of binding to human insulin. The immunoglobulin fraction of the mouse blood can be extracted and will contain the required anti-insulin. However, this fraction will also contain numerous other antibodies and it would be very difficult to isolate the particular antibody that may be required. Because of the multiplicity of immunoglobulin types in the fraction the term 'polyclonal antibody' is used. This polyclonal antibody may even include different antibodies against insulin, i.e. antibodies reactive to different regions (epitopes) of the insulin molecule.

Antibodies are found in all body fluids including blood, milk and mucous secretions and serve an essential role in the immune system that protects animals from infection or the cytotoxic effects of foreign compounds.

Antibodies will bind with high affinity to an invasive molecule. Normally the binding is to only part of a large molecule (the epitope) and so there may be many different antibodies for a particular compound. Antibodies are valuable because of their very specific recognition and affinity for one compound (the antigen).

3.   The structure of antibodies

A structural representation of an antibody (immunoglobulin, IgG) based upon X-ray crystallographic data is shown in *Figure 8.1*. This has an overall molecular mass of 150 kDa and is the major class of immunoglobulin found in blood serum. The molecular structure consists of two light and two heavy chains bound by disulfide bridges. The heavy chain of IgG has four domains VH–CH1–CH2–CH3 and the light chain has two domains VL–CL. The 'constant' region (C) of a particular immunoglobulin class varies only with the species of origin. For example, a human IgG would have a different constant region from a mouse IgG. The variable domains (V) account for the diversity of antibody structure. Digestion of the molecule with papain cleaves the heavy chain in the 'hinge' region and results in three fragments. Two Fab (antibody-binding fragments) each contain the N-terminal end of a heavy chain with disulfide-linked light chain. The other fragment is the Fc which consists of the C-terminal end of the two heavy chains. There are two glycan structures present in the space between the two CH2 domains. In some immunoglobulins there are also glycans present in the variable region of the molecule.

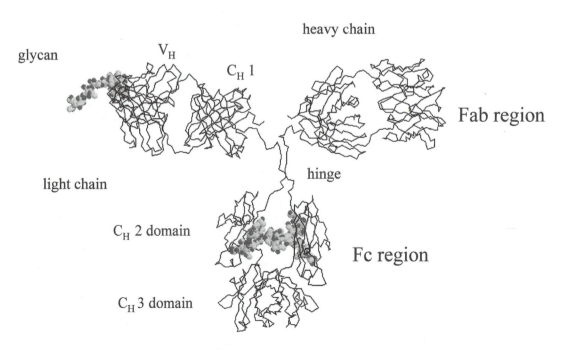

Figure 8.1

Antibody structure – IgG based on X-ray crystallography data. (Figure kindly supplied by Max Crispin.)

Each immunoglobulin molecule has a unique antigen-binding region which consists of hypervariable sequences of amino acids. This region enables the immunoglobulin to bind to one specific molecule (the antigen) with high affinity. The unique antigen-binding site which consists of hypervariable sequences of amino acids is the Fab region. These are formed from three hypervariable loops (complementarity determining regions, CDR) of the VH domain and three hypervariable loops of the VL domain. The variable sequence is produced by somatic recombination and by mutagenesis and accounts for the diversity of antibody molecules. This region enables the antibody to bind to one specific molecule (called the antigen) with high affinity. The other important functional component of the molecule is the effector site which is found in the constant region. The effector functions can be mediated by the Fc region binding to complement (C1q) and to receptors of specific cells. Complement activation leads to the activation of leukocytes and phagocytosis. The Fc receptors are on certain cells of the immune system such as phagocytes and natural killer (NK) cells. Binding to receptors in these cells produces a variety of biological responses including antibody-dependent cellular cytotoxicity (ADCC), phagocytosis, endocytosis and release of inflammatory agents.

4.   Glycosylation of antibodies

Antibodies are glycoproteins containing variable glycan structures (Fukuta *et al.*, 2000). A single conserved N-glycan site is contained in IgG on each CH2 domain of the Fc region at Asn-297 (*Figure 8.1*). The carbohydrate is of a biantennary complex type. The structural variability is associated with a bisected GlcNAc (+/−), core fucosylation (+/−), non-, mono- or digalactosylation and possible sialylation. The glycosylation of the Fc region is essential for effector functions of the antibody such as complement binding, binding to Fc receptors, induction of ADCC and the half-life in the circulatory system. Around 20% of human antibodies are also glycosylated in the variable region of the Fab fragment. This glycan may be important for antigen binding with specific examples showing that the degree of binding may either increase or decrease.

Although the level of glycosylation of IgG is small (2–3% by weight) compared to other proteins, the glycan structures on immunoglobulins are known to have a significant effect on immune responses. *Figure 8.2* shows the common glycoforms of IgG with 0, 1 or 2 galactose terminal residues (G0, G1 and G2) and the possibility of a sialic acid terminal group on G2. The distribution of these glycoforms changes under certain pathological conditions. For example, it is well established that a high proportion of agalactosylated glycan structures in immunoglobulin (G0) is associated with specific human disorders, notably rheumatoid arthritis. Here the predominant form of the glycan attached to Asn-297 is a biantennary complex structure that terminates in N-acetylglucosamine residues and lacks the usual galactose terminus. This altered glycan structure results in a change in the interaction of the immunoglobulin with specific monocyte receptors. Also, there are changes to the structure of the immunoglobulin caused by the altered glycan that may explain changes in immune response related to the disease condition.

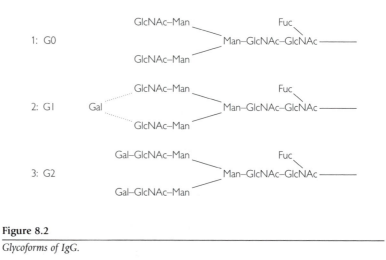

Figure 8.2

Glycoforms of IgG.

5.   Monoclonal antibodies

In the 1970s methods were developed to produce antibodies from cells in culture. In 1975 Kohler and Milstein described a technique to produce cells which were hybrids of B-lymphocytes and myelomas and which were capable of continuous synthesis of preselected antibodies (Kohler and Milstein, 1975). Myeloma cells are transformed lymphocytes capable of growing indefinitely. Since the 1970s, their method has found wide application and has resulted in the large-scale production of kilogram quantities of some monoclonal antibodies. The term 'monoclonal' indicates that the antibody is of a single type, i.e. will bind to just one antigen. Kohler and Milstein obtained the Nobel Prize in 1984 for their work on the development of Mab-secreting hybridomas.

6.   Hybridomas

Hybridomas are hybrid cells capable of the continuous production of mono-clonal antibodies. They combine the key properties of the two parental cells: a myeloma with an infinite lifespan and a B-lymphocyte capable of synthe-sizing a single antibody. Hybridomas can be grown in suspension in large bioreactors for the production of kilogram quantities of monoclonal anti-bodies. The antibodies have a range of applications because of their high specificity in recognizing selected proteins. This enables them to be used for diagnosis and testing in applications such as blood typing, the detection of virus, pregnancy testing or for the detection of contaminants in food. The application of monoclonal antibodies as human therapeutic agents in the treatment of disease has been suggested for a number of years (James, 1990). However, there have been difficulties in the production of antibodies that are not immunogenic to humans. In the late 1990s a range of human or 'humanized' antibodies have been produced specifically for the treatment of cancer. The number of such therapeutic monoclonal antibodies is likely to increase in the future as a result of the numerous clinical trials that are now taking place.

The original work of Kohler and Milstein described the creation of a mouse–mouse hybridoma that secreted antibody with affinity to sheep red blood cells as antigens. The antibody could be easily detected by a hemolytic plaque assay that showed the capability of the antibody to bind to and lyse sheep erythrocytes. Since the 1970s, these methods have found wide application and have resulted in the large-scale production of kilogram quantities of some monoclonal antibodies. The term 'monoclonal' indicates that the antibody is of a single type. This will bind to just one antigen.

The method developed by Kohler and Milstein involves four stages which result in the production of a hybrid lymphocyte with an infinite growth capacity and capable of continuous synthesis of a single antibody. The stages of this process are shown in *Figure 8.3* and involve:

- immunization;
- cell fusion;
- genetic selection;
- cell selection.

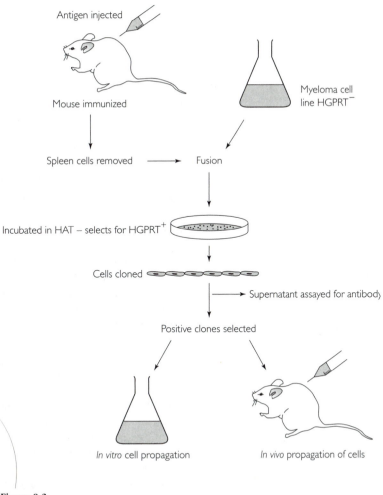

Figure 8.3

Isolation of Mab-secreting hybridomas.

6.1 Immunization *in vivo*

The first stage of the production of a hybridoma is to obtain lymphocytes from an animal that is enriched with specific antibody-secreting cells. Immunization involves the injection of a chosen antigen into an animal – mice and rats have been most commonly used. The time required to produce an immune response resulting in antibody synthesis will depend upon the antigen, but a period of up to 3–4 weeks ensures maximum response. Large molecules tend to produce a strong response over a short period of time. Small molecules are often conjugated to carrier proteins such as albumin and multiple injections spaced over several days may be necessary to enhance the immune response.

Antibodies are synthesized by B-lymphocytes which can be isolated from the spleen of an immunized animal. The isolated spleen is homogenized gently and the lymphocyte cell fraction collected by centrifugation. At this stage the cell fraction is a mixed population with a limited capacity for growth. Approximately 1% of the cell population isolated from the spleen will secrete antibodies.

6.2 Immunization *in vitro*

Although most laboratories use mice for producing active lymphocytes, an alternative approach involves immunization *in vitro* (Borrebaeck, 1988). This process involves the activation of cells obtained from the spleen of a nonimmunized mouse. The cells should be suspended in a medium containing the selected antigen along with various factors stimulating growth and differentiation. These factors can be supplied from culture medium following incubation with mixed lymphocytes (or thymocytes). This is called 'conditioned' medium and contains various growth-promoting factors secreted by the cells. These factors are called cytokines and include interleukins, B-cell growth factor and B-cell differentiation factor. Some of these cytokines have now been well defined and are available as recombinant proteins from commercial suppliers. The effectiveness of immunization *in vitro* is dependent upon the optimal combination of these factors during cell activation.

An advantage of immunization *in vitro* is that the activation of B-lymphocytes takes 3–4 days rather than a few weeks as is the case with immunization *in vivo*. Furthermore, weak antigens at low concentrations can be used. A disadvantage is that certain immunoglobulin isotypes tend to be produced preferentially (usually IgM) although refinement of the techniques during cell activation can stimulate the production of other isotypes.

6.3 Cell hybridization – the process of fusion

In 1965 Harris and Watkins reported that inactivated Sendai virus caused the hybridization of a mixed population of human HeLa cells and mouse Ehrlich ascites tumor cells (Harris and Watkins, 1965). The result of the fusion was a mixed population of hybrid cells (called heterokaryons) that were genetically unstable. *Figure 8.4* indicates the sequence of events during fusion showing the cytoplasmic fusion of two dissimilar cells followed by the hybridization of the nuclei of the two cells. After a period of growth the heterokaryons tend to lose some of their genetic material and become stable

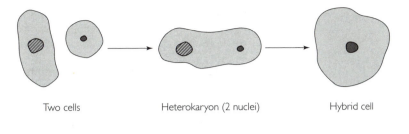

Two cells   Heterokaryon (2 nuclei)   Hybrid cell

Figure 8.4

Cell hybridization.

hybrids retaining some of the phenotypic characteristics of each parental cell. The method turned out to be an extremely valuable tool for biological research, particularly in developing an understanding of gene regulation. In 1969 Harris showed that when normal cells were fused with malignant cells the malignant phenotype was not always retained. This was the first direct evidence for the existence of human suppressor genes, derived from the normal cells and that could result in suppression of the tumorigenic characteristics. These genes, whose products include the retinoblastoma protein and p53, are now well characterized in terms of their role in malignancies.

Cell fusion has also been used extensively in human chromosome mapping. The heterokaryons resulting from the fusion of human and mouse cells are genetically unstable and tend to lose human chromosomes randomly. This eventually gives rise to a mixed population of stable hybrids from which individual cell clones can be isolated. Many of these clones may contain single human chromosomes. It is the association of a particular chromosome in an isolated cell clone with a selected measurable phenotypic characteristic such as an enzyme activity that allows the gene of that enzyme to be assigned to a specific human chromosome. With the use of this technique, many human genes have been assigned to particular chromosomes (known as 'chromosome mapping').

It was this same technique of cell fusion that Kohler and Milstein used in their work reported in 1975 that allowed the creation of stable hybrid cells from the hybridization of antibody-secreting B-lymphocytes with transformed myelomas. The resulting cells retained two important phenotypic characteristics from the parents – the ability for infinite growth (from the myeloma) and the ability to synthesize antibody (from the lymphocyte). The original objective of this work was to study somatic mutation as a mechanism for antibody diversity. This is the ability of B-lymphocytes to go through a maturation process following initial contact with an antigen to produce antibodies of increasing affinity. However, the application of the cell fusion technique to produce antibody-producing cells with an infinite growth capacity had a major impact on the ability to produce large quantities of antibodies that could be used for a variety of functions both in biological research and also as medically important products. The term 'hybridoma' was derived in 1976 by Herzenberg and Milstein to describe a homogeneous clone of these antibody-producing hybrid cells. The term 'monoclonal antibody' refers to the secreted product of the cells. Unlike antibodies derived from blood samples ('polyclonal'), the monoclonal antibodies from a single hybridoma are molecularly homogeneous, all having an identical molecular structure and a specific affinity for a particular antigen.

6.4 Cell fusion to immortalize lymphocytes

Although immunization can result in lymphocytes capable of producing the required antibody, the cells will only grow for a limited period of time. The purpose of lymphocyte hybridization is to combine the desired property of antibody synthesis of the B-lymphocyte population with the infinite growth capacity of a myeloma. Therefore, the selected lymphocytes are fused with a population of myeloma cells. Those commonly used for mouse or rat cells are shown in *Table 8.1*. Suitable myeloma fusion partners are selected for two other important characteristics:

■ nonproduction of antibodies. This is desirable so that the resulting hybridoma does not synthesize more than one antibody;

■ possession of a genetic marker, such as the lack of an enzyme, to allow cell selection. For example, myelomas deficient in HGPRT (hypoxanthine guanine phosphoribosyl transferase) are commonly used. This allows selection of hybridomas in HAT (hypoxanthine, aminopterin, thymidine) medium (see Section 6.6).

To allow fusion the activated B-lymphocytes are mixed with a suitable fusion partner – the myeloma.

6.5 Methods of cell fusion

Cells can be induced to fuse if two cell populations are brought close together at a high cell concentration (10^6 to 10^7 cells per well of a 96 multi-well plate) in the presence of viruses or by chemical agents (called 'fusogens'). The process involves the destabilization of adjacent cell membranes which eventually fuse to form a hybrid cell. Initially, two distinct nuclei are present in the fused cell (a heterokaryon). Eventually the nuclei fuse to produce a stable hybrid cell.

Although UV-inactivated Sendai viruses were originally used as agents for cell fusion, the more widely used method is now fusion by the chemical agent polyethylene glycol (PEG). This is a polymer, available at a molecular weight range of 200–20 000 kDa. PEG at 4000–6000 kDa is most suitable for cell fusion. Cell fusion can occur in a solution of PEG (40–50% w/v) within 1–2 minutes. In this process, cell swelling accompanies fusion. This

Table 8.1. Commonly used rodent cell lines (myelomas) as fusion partners

Species	Cell line	Immunoglobulin expression
Mouse	X653	No
	NS0	No
	Sp2/0	No
	NSI	Yes
Rat	YB2/0	No
	Y3-Ag	Yes

enables adjacent cells to approach very closely and also the plasma membrane becomes permeable to small ions. However, lysis of swollen cells may also occur.

Alternatively, electrofusion can be used. In this technique, two populations of cells are introduced into a small sterile chamber. An electric current is applied in high-voltage pulses for short time periods. During this period the membrane will become highly permeable. This is similar to the process of electroporation used to facilitate the entry of DNA into cells. This causes the cells to orientate along the line of the current and fuse. This process is highly efficient, producing a high percentage of viable hybrid cells. The most suitable voltage for electrofusion is one that causes approximately 50% death in the cell population. This would typically be around a voltage of 200 V for a cell pellet held in a small electroporation cuvette. From such a protocol there may be around 50 fused cells from an original total of 5×10^6 cells from each parental cell line.

6.6 Selectable gene markers for cell selection

The process of cell fusion will result in a heterogeneous population of cells that will contain unfused parental cells, lysed cells as well as the required hybrid cells. At this stage, cell selection is important so that the hybrid cells can be isolated from the mixture. For hybridomas there are two important stages of cell selection:

■   isolation of hybrid cells from parental cells;
■   selection of antibody-secreting cells within the hybrid cell population.

The basis of cell selection is to distinguish cell types through genetic differences. One required characteristic of the resulting hybridomas is the ability for effective growth in culture. So, initial cell selection can involve the incubation of the mixed population of cells in a suitable culture environment. This includes the addition of a suitable liquid growth medium to the cells and incubation at 37°C for a few days. This will allow the growth of all viable cells which will include the hybridomas and myelomas. Growth of these cells will dilute any nonviable and lysed cells from the mixture. Unfused lymphocytes have only a limited capacity for growth and will be eliminated eventually.

The hybridomas are selected from the myelomas on the basis of a genetic marker that is normally applied to the myelomas. The most commonly used genetic marker is HGPRT⁻ which indicates a cell with a defective enzyme, hypoxanthine guanine phosphoribosyl transferase. This is a normal metabolic enzyme that is capable of catalyzing the addition of phosphoribosyl pyrophosphate on to hypoxanthine or guanine. This constitutes the salvage pathway for converting purines to nucleotides as part of nucleotide synthesis in all normal cells (*Figure 8.5*). However, there is an alternative pathway of nucleotide formation which involves the complete synthesis of the purine ring (called the '*de novo*' pathway) from smaller metabolic precursors. Normal cells can utilize either pathway depending upon the nutrient precursors available in the surrounding media.

The myelomas chosen for cell hybridization with lymphocytes have an HGPRT⁻ genetic marker through previous random mutation and selection. However, the hybridomas would be expected to have normal HGPRT activity

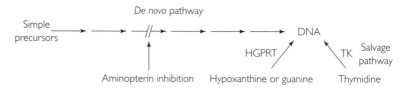

Figure 8.5

De novo *and salvage pathways of nucleotide synthesis.*

(HGPRT$^+$) because they receive the normal gene from the parental lymph-ocyte. Either cell line would be able to grow normally in cell culture medium in which standard nutrients are provided. The *de novo* pathway for nucleotide synthesis would operate in both cells, although the salvage pathway would only occur in the hybridomas.

The principle of selection is to place these cells into a 'selective medium' in which the *de novo* pathway of nucleotide synthesis is inhibited. The key to this is the compound, aminopterin, which is an analog of folic acid and a specific inhibitor of dihydrofolate reductase, an essential enzyme for the for-mation of tetrahydrofolate (FH$_4$) required as a co-enzyme of the *de novo* purine nucleotide synthesis pathway. Tetrahydrofolate is also required for the formation of thymidine. However, if hypoxanthine and thymidine are provided in the culture media of HGPRT$^+$ cells they will be able to grow nor-mally. On the other hand HGPRT$^-$ cells have no means of synthesizing purine nucleotides and consequently would be unable to grow.

The selective medium HAT contains hypoxanthine, aminopterin and thymidine. This medium allows the selection and growth of hybridomas which are HGPRT$^+$ and have a normal functioning salvage pathway. However, HAT is unable to support the growth of the HGPRT$^-$ myelomas because the *de novo* pathway is inhibited and the salvage pathway cannot function because of the defective enzyme.

In the mixed population of cells resulting from fusion, the newly formed hybridomas will be HGPRT$^+$ by inheritance from normal lymphocytes whereas the unfused myelomas carry the mutant HGPRT$^-$ marker. Therefore incubation in HAT will allow survival of the HGPRT$^+$ hybridomas but not the HGPRT$^-$ myelomas. So, after a few days incubation in HAT the culture will contain only hybridomas.

6.7   Clonal selection of Mab-secreting hybridomas

After genetic selection with HAT the culture contains hybridomas but only some of these will secrete antibodies. Although the efficiencies of synthesis vary considerably, only about 10% of the population of hybridomas formed from cell fusion would be expected to secrete antibody. The next stage involves selection of Mab-secreting hybridomas from the population which has survived HAT treatment. Cell clones can be isolated by the method of limiting dilution. Cloning ensures that all cells selected for future cultures are genetically identical. This involves dispensing a cell suspension into a 96-well plate, so that each well contains an average of one cell.

Hybridomas grow poorly at low densities but growth can be supported by a feeder layer of cells. This consists of a population of cells (e.g. thymocytes, macrophages or splenocytes) which have been treated to prevent any growth. The treatment may be by gamma irradiation or exposure to mitomycin C which halts DNA synthesis. Typically cells would be treated with 10 µg/ml mitomycin C for 2 h at 37°C. Under these conditions the cellular metabolism continues and secreted growth factors can promote the growth of viable hybridoma cells particularly if they are inoculated at low density. Feeder layers can be purchased as frozen suspensions.

After allowing 1–2 weeks for growth, the medium of each well should be tested for antibody content using a suitable assay. Wells containing a high antibody titer are then selected for further cell growth. At this stage the cells may be genetically unstable and a second round of cloning is recommended to ensure the isolation of a stable population of high-level antibody-secreting cells. This involves further testing of the culture medium for antibody content.

Antibody-secreting hybridomas can be grown in culture in suspension to produce $1-2 \times 10^6$ cells/ml and a Mab concentration of 100–200 µg/ml (*Figure 8.6*). The cells can generally be adapted to serum-free medium while maintaining high productivity.

7.   Assay of monoclonal antibodies

There are three assay procedures that are commonly used to detect monoclonal antibodies in solution. Each is suitable for the measurement of Mab concentration in culture media.

■   ELISA – enzyme-linked immunosorbent assay.
■   RIA – radioimmunoassay.
■   Affinity chromatography.

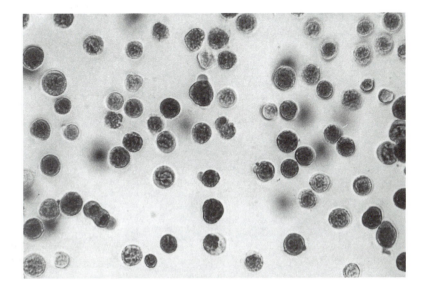

Figure 8.6

Hybridomas in suspension during exponential growth.

ELISA is the most commonly used assay for antibodies and is adapted to multi-well plates for analyzing multiple samples. RIA is more sensitive but is more time consuming and expensive. Affinity chromatography is ideal if an HPLC system is available and the hybridomas are growing in a serum-free medium. The basis of the three types of assay are described here.

7.1 Enzyme-linked immunosorbent assay (ELISA)

This is a solid phase binding assay that can easily be performed in a 96–well plate (*Figure 8.7*). ELISA measures antigen or antibody concentration, depending on the protocol used. The stages of a typical assay involve a series of additions in which each component binds to the one previously added.

- An appropriate antigen is bound to the plastic of the base of the plate. Most large proteins bind spontaneously. Difficulties with binding of small molecular weight antigens can be overcome by forming a conjugate with a larger molecule such as bovine serum albumin (BSA).
- The remaining attachment sites are blocked on the solid support by addition of a non-interfering protein such as BSA.
- A solution of the Mab under test or a standard antibody solution is added. This will bind to the antigen held on the solid support.
- An antibody–enzyme conjugate with specificity against the first antibody is added. The second antibody is species specific. This means that it binds to any immunoglobulin of the species from which the first antibody is derived, e.g. goat anti-mouse antibody. An enzyme such as alkaline phosphatase is conjugated to the second antibody which can then be detected by a colorimetric assay. Conjugated anti-Ig antibodies are available commercially.

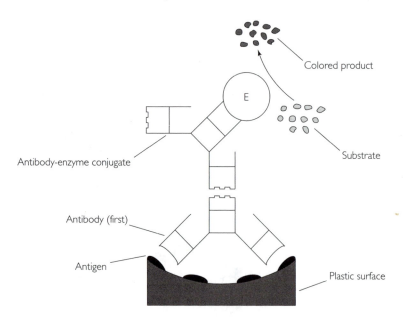

Figure 8.7

Enzyme-linked immunosorbent assay (ELISA).

■ Finally a suitable enzyme substrate is added. The substrate is one which can be changed to a colored product by the enzyme bound to the conjugate. For example, p-nitrophenyl phosphate would be suitable for an alkaline phosphatase conjugate. The extent of coloration in each well of a plate can be measured by a multi-well reader.

7.2 Radioimmunoassay (RIA)

A solid phase binding assay similar to ELISA can be adapted to radioactive detection when a radioactively labeled antigen or antibody is used. The RIA is more sensitive and reliable than ELISA but is usually more time consuming and more expensive because of the cost of the radioactive label.

7.3 Affinity binding

Certain bacterial cell wall proteins (called Protein A and Protein G) bind with high affinity to mammalian immunoglobulins. Protein A is derived from *Staphylococcus aureus* and has a strong affinity for antibodies. This allows antibodies to be isolated by chromatography columns which contain inert beads conjugated to Protein A or G. If a sample (such as Mab-containing culture medium) is run through the column at neutral pH only antibodies will bind, allowing all other components to be washed out. Pure antibody can then be eluted from the column by a low pH buffer.

Suitable affinity columns of this type have been designed for use with high-performance liquid chromatography (HPLC) and this offers an extremely rapid method of analyzing or purifying antibodies. However, the method will detect any mammalian immunoglobulin which means that the immunoglobulin content of the serum used in the growth medium may interfere with analysis.

HPLC affinity columns (such as ProAnaMabs from Hyclone) offer a rapid assay for measuring antibodies in serum-free culture medium and they could be used instead of ELISA. Affinity chromatography can also be used for large-scale antibody extraction, although the preparative Protein A or G columns are expensive.

8. Human monoclonal antibodies

Although murine-derived monoclonal antibodies are widely used as laboratory reagents, in affinity purification and clinical diagnostic tests, they have had limited success in human therapy. Immunoglobulins synthesized from mice and humans have different constant regions and so any antibody of mouse origin injected into a human could elicit an undesirable immune reaction. Firstly, although the antigen-binding site might be appropriate for the target, the antibody will not produce appropriate human effector responses such as those of complement and Fc receptor binding. Secondly, the human immune system will produce antibodies against the murine immunoglobulin. This is referred to as the human anti-murine antibody (HAMA) immune response.

This presents an obstacle in developing therapeutic antibodies from a murine source. However, there are at least three major difficulties in producing human hybridoma cells capable of secreting human monoclonal antibodies.

8.1 The source of antibody-secreting lymphocytes

In generating murine hybridomas, the spleen of an immunized mouse is used as a source of the mixed lymphocyte population for cell selection. Clearly this is not possible with humans and the source of human lymphocytes is limited to samples of peripheral blood. These can be taken from patients who have acquired an immunity against a particular compound or disease. Alternatively, methods of *in vitro* immunization of human lymphocytes are possible. This approach requires the optimization of conditions for human B-lymphocyte activation by use of the appropriate cytokines and growth factors.

8.2 Immortalization and chromosome instability

There must be a suitable human fusion partner to immortalize the B-lymphocytes. Human myeloma cell lines are difficult to grow in culture. Human lymphoblastoid cell lines have been used as fusion partners but the frequency of cell fusion and genetic stability of the resulting hybridomas is low compared with equivalent fusions with mouse cells. An alternative approach is to immortalize the activated human lymphocytes by transfection with oncogenic DNA or by transformation by a virus.

8.3 Antibody secretion of human parental fusion partners

Mouse myelomas commonly used in fusion are nonantibody secretors. The value of this is that the resulting hybridomas only secrete the antibody associated with the fused B-lymphocyte. Therefore, the culture product will be a single selected antibody type. However, most of the human myeloma or lymphoblastoid cells commonly used for hybridization are immunoglobulin secretors (*Table 8.2*). This means that the resulting selected human hybridoma will secrete at least two antibodies, which are those associated with each of the parental cells.

9. Recombinant antibodies

A further possibility is the humanization of monoclonal antibodies originally produced from mice. This process involves antibody engineering, which relies on the techniques of recombinant DNA technology to re-arrange some of the molecular domains of an immunoglobulin (Hudson and Souriau, 2003). Examples of these are shown in *Figure 8.8*. In a chimeric

Table 8.2. Human or human hybrid fusion partners

Cell type	Cell line	Immunoglobulin expression
Human myeloma	SK007	Yes
Human lymphoblastoid	RH-L4	Yes but nonsecretor
Human lymphoblastoid	GM1500	Yes
Human lymphoblastoid	KR4	Yes
Human lymphoblastoid	LICR-LON	Yes
Human/human hybridoma	KR12	Yes
Human/mouse hybridoma	SHM-D33	Yes but nonsecretor

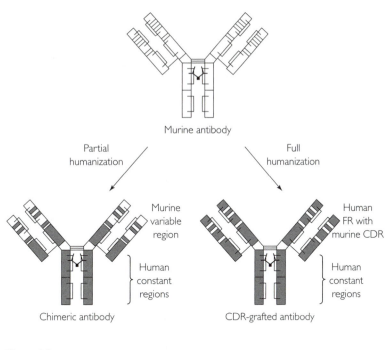

Figure 8.8

Ways to humanize an antibody.

antibody the mouse variable regions are linked to human constant regions. Thus in such a construct the antigen-binding site of the murine antibody is retained but the human constant region contributes the immunogenicity through the effector functions. A further step to humanizing the antibody is by replacing portions of the V-region that are not required for the antigen-binding site. The framework regions (FR residues) which were originally murine are replaced by human regions. Thus only the complementarity-determining regions (CDRs) are retained as of murine origin. Hybrid antibodies of this type have now been used as human therapeutic agents.

The elimination of the murine constant regions reduces the previously experienced HAMA response. It is not always certain that complete humanization has an advantage over a chimeric antibody because humanization of the V-region may result in a loss in affinity to the antigen. Also, it is not clear that the problem of unwanted immunogenicity can be totally removed because repeated doses of even a fully humanized antibody may elicit an anti-idiotype response, that is directed against the antigen-binding site. However, these developments in humanized therapeutic antibodies have allowed the introduction of a range of products against specific human diseases (*Table 8.3*).

9.1 Recombinant antibody fragments

Various fragments of human immunoglobulins have been expressed successfully in bacterial cells. These include the Fv fragment, the single-chain Fv fragment (scFv), the Fab fragment and the F(ab)2 fragment (*Figure 8.9*). The Fv is the smallest antigen-binding fragment of an immunoglobulin with a

Table 8.3. Examples of Mabs approved for human therapy

Commercial name	Type of Mab	Therapeutic use	Year approved
Orthoclone, OKT3	Murine	Allograft/rejection	1986
ReoPro	Chimeric	Angioplasty	1994
Rituxan	Chimeric	Non-Hodgkin's lymphoma	1997
Herceptin	CDR-grafted	Breast cancer	1998
Zenapax	CDR-grafted	Transplant rejection	1997
Simulect	Chimeric	Transplant rejection	1998
Remicade	Chimeric	Rheumatoid arthritis and Crohn's disease	1998
Synagis	CDR-grafted	Respiratory syncytial virus (RSV)	1998
Mylotarg	CDR-grafted	Acute myeloid leukemia	2001
Campath	CDR-grafted	Chronic lymphocytic leukemia	2001
Humira	Human	Modifying antirheumatic drugs	2002

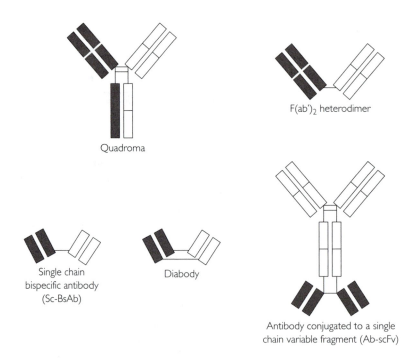

Figure 8.9

Recombinant antibody fragments.

molecular mass of around 25 kDa. The VH and VL domains of the Fv fragment are stabilized by disulfide bridges. In the scFv fragment a short peptide spacer (usually 15–20 amino acids) is introduced in order to link the VH and VL domains covalently. This also allows the possibility of the linkage of two scFv fragments to create 'diabodies' which are bispecific in so far as they have two independent antigen-binding sites. Bispecific antibodies can also be produced from the fusion of two hybridomas to generate a 'quadroma'.

However, all combinations of light and heavy chains are synthesized in these cells with only a few of the molecules being bispecific. Purification of the required molecules would be a difficult task.

The potential advantage of these recombinant fragments for human therapy is their small size that facilitates tissue penetration, biodistribution and blood clearance. The fragments can be isolated from libraries of antibodies displayed on the surface of filamentous bacteriophages. This phage display technology is an alternative strategy that can be used instead of mammalian hybridoma technology. The disadvantage is that the recombinant antibody fragments lack glycosylation and also the binding sites for complement and Fc receptors. However, the possibilities exist of conjugating other polypeptide sequences to express the desired effector functions. Conjugation of toxins or specific growth factors to these fragments also allows the future development of immuno-constructs with considerable potential for therapeutic activity.

10. Potential alternative methods of production

10.1 Antibodies from plants

Antibodies were first expressed in transgenic plants in 1989 (Hiatt *et al.*, 1989). Since then various antibody fragments and domains have been produced in plant hosts as well as full-length and multimeric antibodies. The most popular host species for this work has been the tobacco plant, *Nicotiana*, although corn and soybeans have also been utilized. There is no apparent reason why other plants could not be used (Ma and Hein, 1995). The value of using plants for monoclonal antibody production includes the absence of animal pathogens, the ease of genetic manipulation, the ability of post-translational modification and the potential for scale-up to an economic production process.

Transformation involves the stable integration of the appropriate DNA into the plant cell genome. The resulting transgenic plants can be cross-fertilized so as to integrate the genes of a multimeric protein structure in a single genetically stable hybrid plant. One major advantage of monoclonal antibodies from plants is the potential low cost of large-scale production. These so called 'plantibodies' can be produced at an estimated cost of $0.01 to $0.1 per milligram as opposed to $1 to $5 per milligram for production from cell culture processing of animal-derived hybridomas. The cost of microbial fermentation is lower than that of mammalian cell culture but bacteria lack the ability for efficient multimeric protein assembly and of any post-translational modification. A further potential advantage of the plantibodies is delivery by consumption of plant tissue and thus avoiding any need for purification. These possibilities are particularly applicable in certain cases such as the previously shown ability of a plant-produced antibody against *Streptococcus mutans* to prevent binding of the bacteria to the surface of teeth, thus reducing tooth decay (Verch *et al.*, 1998).

Plant cells are eukaryotes and therefore capable of post-translational modification of proteins including N-linked glycosylation. However, although the plant glycan structures have not been analyzed in detail it is likely that these structures are significantly different from those in mammalian systems. For example, the commonly found mammalian terminal sialic acid (N-acetyl neuraminic acid) residue is a structure not found in plants. Also the α-1,3 core fucose structure appears to be unique to plants and has been implicated in human allergies to pollen. The potential presence of such unusual glycan structures in plant-derived antibodies might not have an effect on antigen binding but for a therapeutic antibody they are likely to increase the chance of an adverse immunogenic reaction during human treatment. This could limit the use of plant-derived antibodies in certain applications particularly if systemic long-term administration is required.

10.2   Humanized antibodies from transgenic mice

Transgenic mice strains have been produced capable of synthesizing human monoclonal antibodies. Xenomouse strains have large portions of human variable region genes incorporated into the germ line via a yeast artificial chromosome (YAC). The megabase-sized YAC allows the genes for human heavy and light chain immunoglobulin to be incorporated as transgenes into a mouse strain deficient in the production of murine Ig. The large human variable region repertoire incorporated as transgenes allows the mice to generate a diverse immune response comparable to that in humans. These human genes are also compatible with the mouse enzymes that allow class switching from IgM to IgG. The immunoglobulin generation will also undergo somatic hypermutation and affinity maturation, a natural process that enhances the affinity of the antibody for the antigen. Thus an antigen introduced into a Xenomouse produces a human monoclonal antibody with high specificity for its corresponding antigen. Such antibodies have already proved their potential in clinical trials.

11.   The importance of glycosylation to therapeutic antibodies

The glycosylation pattern of the immunoglobulin structure has particular relevance to the production and use of monoclonal antibodies as therapeutic agents. Any *in vitro* production process results in a heterogeneity of glycan structures of the product protein. To avoid any undesirable immune response in the use of such antibodies it is important to maximize the content of fully processed glycans. There are various parameters that affect the glycan processing from the metabolic profile of the hybridoma to the environmental conditions of culture. It has been shown that the glycan structures vary with the specific activity of key glycosylating enzymes contained in a hybridoma. This in turn depends upon the enzymic profile of the parental cell lines used in the hybridization process. In one study hybridomas were produced from parental cell lines, only one of which had an enzyme (UDP-N-acetylglucosamine: β-D-mannoside β-1,4-N-acetylglucosaminyltransferase; GnT III) responsible for the addition of a bisecting GlcNAc. As expected the resulting hybridomas had varying levels of GnT III. Of interest was the fact that the content of bisecting GlcNAc in the antibodies produced by each hybridoma was a reflection of the intracellular activity of GnT III.

A further example of the effect of the producer cell line on the glycosylation pattern of a monoclonal antibody has been shown for the IgG,

CAMPATH-1H. This is a humanized recombinant murine monoclonal antibody developed for human therapy and has been expressed in various cell lines including a murine myeloma and Chinese hamster ovary (CHO). The glycosylation of the antibody produced from CHO was consistent with normal human IgG. That is fucosylated biantennary structures containing zero, one or two galactose residues. However, the immunoglobulin from a murine myeloma (NS0) results in some potentially immunogenic glycoforms containing Galα(1–3)Gal terminal residues. Such hypergalactosylated proteins have been shown following expression from various murine cells.

Cell culture conditions have also been shown to affect product glycosylation. Relevant culture parameters include the accumulation of ammonia, the dissolved oxygen level, glucose depletion, lipid composition, pH and protein content of the medium. The glycosylation of monoclonal antibodies from hybridomas is particularly susceptible to the dissolved oxygen level of the culture, which on a large scale is often maintained at a specific setpoint through an oxygen probe that controls the gaseous input to the bioreactor. This dissolved oxygen (DO) is usually calibrated from 0 to 100%, which is the level of oxygen relative to saturation with air. The relative proportion of three predominant glycoforms (*Figure 8.2*) changes depending upon culture conditions. For example, the dissolved oxygen level of a hybridoma culture has a noticeable effect on this distribution. Whereas a normal distribution of G0, G1 and G2 is found at 50% DO, lower levels of oxygen (<10%) may lead to poor galactosylation and a consequent increased proportion of G0.

12. Conclusion

The ability to produce monoclonal antibodies from hybridomas emerged from a technology developed in the early 1970s and reported in 1975. Since then monoclonal antibodies have found wide application in research and in diagnostic tests because of their high specificity in recognizing antigens. However, the therapeutic application of monoclonal antibodies has taken a long time because of a range of side-effects associated with undesirable immune responses in humans of murine-derived antibodies. The situation is now rapidly changing with the ability to produce humanized or fully human antibodies. This has enabled the approval of monoclonal antibodies for a range of therapies including transplantation, cancer, infectious disease, cardiovascular disease and inflammation. There are many antibodies approved by the FDA for therapeutic use (see *Table 8.3*) with several hundred awaiting the results of clinical trial. Because these approved antibodies are human (or humanized) immunoglobulins they enable effector functions to direct complement-dependent cytotoxicity to a target cell. Other biological effects are also possible by conjugation of compounds to the antibody.

Therapeutic antibodies are required in much larger quantities than those used in diagnosis or as laboratory reagents. Therefore it is certain that the requirements for large-scale production of hybridomas will increase. There is a need to ensure that the conditions of culture are compatible with full and appropriate human glycosylation profiles of the synthesized immunoglobulins. Therefore work to understand fully those conditions that allow this to take place will continue.

References

Borrebaeck, C.A.K. (ed.) (1988) *In Vitro Immunization in Hybridoma Technology.* Elsevier, Amsterdam.

Fukuta, K., Abe R., Yokomatsu, T., Kono, N., Nagatomi, Y., Asanagi, M., Shimazaki, Y. and Makino, T. (2000) Comparative study of the N-glycans of human monoclonal immunoglobulins M produced by hybridoma and parental cells. *Arch. Biochem. Biophys.* **378**: 142–150.

Harris, H. and Watkins, J.F. (1965) Hybrid cells from mouse and man: Artificial heterokaryons of mammalian cells from different species. *Nature* **205**: 640–646.

Hiatt, A., Cafferkey, R. and Bowdish, K. (1989) Production of antibodies in transgenic plants. *Nature* **342**: 76–78.

Hudson, P.J. and Souriau, C. (2003) Engineered antibodies (Review). *Nat. Med.* **9**: 129–134.

James, K. (1990) Therapeutic monoclonal antibodies – their production and application. In: Spier, R.E. and Griffiths, J.B. (eds) *Animal Cell Biotechnology*, Vol. 4, pp. 205–255. Academic Press, London.

Kohler, G. and Milstein, C. (1975) Continuous cultures of fused cells secreting antibody of predefined specificity. *Nature* **256**: 495–497.

Ma, J.K. and Hein, M.B. (1995) Immunotherapeutic potential of antibodies produced in plants. *Trends Biotechnol.* **13**: 522–527.

Verch, T., Yusibov, V. and Koprowski, H. (1998) Expression and assembly of a full-length monoclonal antibody in plants using a plant virus vector. *J. Immunol. Methods* **220**: 69–75.

Further reading

Borrebaeck, C.A.K. and Hagen, I. (eds) (1993) *Electromanipulation in Hybridoma Technology: A Laboratory Manual.* Stockton Press & W.H.Freeman/OUP, New York.

Cambrosio, A. and Keating, P. (1996) *Exquisite Specificity: The Monoclonal Antibody Revolution.* Oxford University Press, Oxford.

Delves, P.J. (ed.) (1994) *Cellular Immunology Labfax.* Academic Press, London.

Gaerhert, P.J. (2002) The roots of antibody diversity. *Nature* **419**: 29–31.

Harbour, C. and Fletcher, A. (1991) Hybridomas: production and selection. In: Butler, M. (ed.) *Mammalian Cell Biotechnology: A Practical Approach*, pp. 109–138. Oxford University Press, Oxford.

Malik, V.S. and Lillehoj, E.P. (eds) (1994) *Antibody Techniques.* Academic Press, London.

Mather, J. and Barnes, D. (eds) (1998) *Animal Cell Culture Methods.* Academic Press, London.

Maynard, J. and Georgiou, G. (2000) Antibody engineering. *Annu. Rev. Biomed. Eng.* **2**: 339–376.

McCullough, K. and Spier, R.E. (1990) *Monoclonal Antibodies in Biotechnology: Theoretical and Practical Aspects. Cambridge Studies in Biotechnology*, Vol. 8. Cambridge University Press, Cambridge.

Milstein, C. (1980) Monoclonal antibodies. *Sci. Am.* **243**: 66–74.

Mizrahi, A. (ed.) (1989) *Advances in Biotechnological Processes, Vol. 11. Monoclonal Antibodies: Production and Application.* A.R. Liss, New York.

Seaver, S.S. (ed.) (1986) *Commercial Production of Monoclonal Antibodies.* Marcel Dekker, New York.

Springer, T.A. (ed.) (1985) *Hybridoma Technology in the Biosciences and Medicine.* Plenum Press, New York.

Wang, H.Y. and Imanaka, T. (eds) (1999) *Antibody Expression and Engineering.* Oxford University Press, Oxford.

Wentworth, P. Jr. (2002) Antibody design by man and nature. *Science* **296**: 2247–2249.

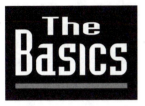

Chapter 9

Scaling up animal cell culture

1. Why scale-up cultures?

Small volume cultures are preferable for experiments requiring a large number of replicates. This might be necessary, for example, in the determination of the concentration-dependent effects of substances that promote or inhibit cell growth. Multi-well plates (e.g. 24-well plates) can accommodate culture volumes of 2–3 ml which are adequate for single determinations of cell concentration which may be taken after a suitable growth period of a few days. If an experiment requires multiple samples to be taken over time to observe cell growth and to perform substrate or product assays, then culture volumes up to 100 ml are usually adequate. Such experiments would normally be conducted in T-flasks or spinner flasks in a temperature-controlled CO_2 incubator (see Chapter 3). Small volume cultures have a large surface area/volume ratio. This allows easy diffusion of gases through the culture surface.

Culture scale-up is required to produce substantial quantities of a cell product, such as a virus or a glycoprotein, or to obtain a sufficient quantity of cells for metabolite or enzyme extraction. There are two approaches to scale-up:

- a multiple process would involve handling 1000 culture flasks (100 ml);
- a unit process would involve a 100-liter fermenter.

Cultures of 1–5 liters are suitable for simulating commercial culture processes in a laboratory because at this scale of operation some parameters that can be ignored in low-volume cultures now become important and need to be controlled. These parameters include the method of oxygen supply, temperature control, pH control and culture mixing. A standard set of electrodes can monitor oxygen, pH and temperature.

To obtain high cell densities and maximum productivity of secreted proteins, the type and design of the bioreactor and mode of operation need to be considered carefully.

2. The stirred tank reactor (STR)

A bioreactor is a term often used instead of a fermenter to describe equipment designed to grow cells in culture. The stirred tank bioreactor (or reactor) is the simplest and most widely used of all fermenter designs and consists of a cylindrical vessel with a stirrer (a pot and paddle). The design has been used extensively in all microbial fermentation and has been the main system used in yeast fermentation in the brewing industry for centuries. However, animal cells are more fragile and grow more slowly than most bacteria or fungi. They require gentler culture conditions and control systems that are optimized for lower metabolic rates. Therefore, the design, mode of operation and control systems of an STR used for animal cells are distinctly different from those that would be applicable to bacterial or fungal cells. This is an important point because attempts at *ad hoc* modifications of a fermenter designed for bacteria are unlikely to be successful in growing animal cells.

The STR has been developed commercially in large-scale animal cell culture processes up to a volume of at least 10 000 liters. For laboratory use there are also numerous bench-top STRs (1–5 liters) that are available commercially and that have been designed specifically for animal cell cultures. Small vessels (<20 liters) are made of glass whereas stainless steel is used for larger ones (>20 liters). *Figure 9.1* shows a typical glass design. Bioreactors like this one with a working volume of about 5 liters can be sterilized by autoclaving with the electrodes in position.

Bench-top models are generally made of glass with a stainless steel head plate, whereas the larger fermenters are made entirely from stainless steel. The metal head plate of an STR consists of a range of ports and pipes. This allows electrodes to be inserted and tubing to be attached for media input or sampling.

Manufacturers of bench-top models include the following: Applikon, New Brunswick, LH Fermentation, Setric SGI, Braun, Bio-engineering. Each of these companies produces uniquely designed and controlled fermenters,

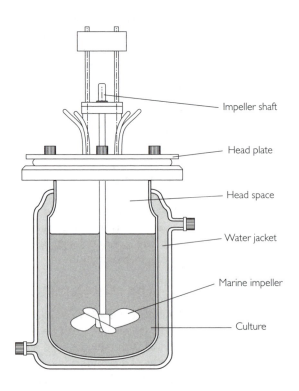

Impeller shaft

Head plate

Head space

Water jacket

Marine impeller

Culture

Figure 9.1

Stirred tank bioreactor.

all of which have been shown to be suitable for animal cell culture. *Figure 9.2* shows the LH 210 bench-top animal cell bioreactor. The vessel (5 liter) at this scale can be made of glass (*Figure 9.3*) whereas at higher volumes stainless steel is used as in the case of the 500-liter stirred bioreactor shown in *Figure 9.4*.

There are several features of STRs that can be utilized to ensure adequate control of culture parameters such as agitation, temperature control, pH control and oxygen supply. These features will be described in this chapter.

2.1 Agitation

The fragility of animal cells in culture has been a subject of considerable interest and debate in relation to fermenter design. Although cells in suspension can be damaged by various forces acting in a stirred culture, the major damaging force is from bubble bursting on the culture surface resulting from culture aeration. The hydrodynamic shear force resulting from the motion of a stirrer is thought to be of lesser importance; nevertheless the stirring speeds commonly adopted for animal cell cultures are considerably lower than those for bacterial cultures of equivalent volume.

The simplest stirring operation involves the rotation of a suspended bar by a magnetic stirrer. This is the system used in glass spinner bottles and is suitable for stirring cultures up to a volume of 1 liter. At larger volumes, such magnetic stirrers are not suitable because of the increased energy required

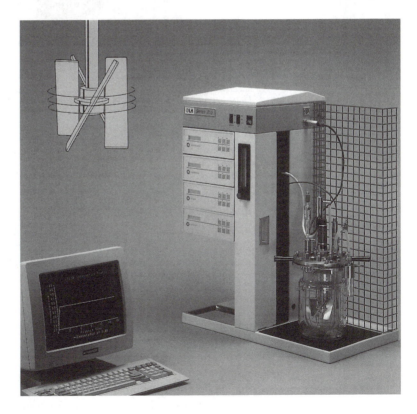

Figure 9.2

Bench-top bioreactor designed for animal cell cultures. Courtesy of LH Fermentation Catalogue

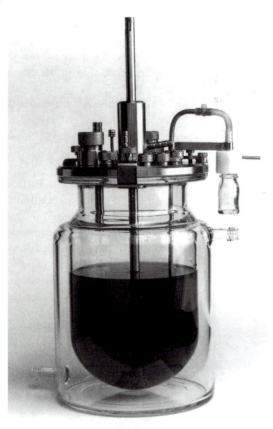

Figure 9.3

Glass bioreactor (5 liter) with stainless steel head plate.

for rotation. Top-drive mechanical motors are normally used for STRs from bench-top models to the larger commercial fermenters. In the design shown in *Figure 9.1* the stirring shaft fits through the stainless steel head plate and into the sterile culture. The stirring motor and outer part of the drive shaft can normally be disconnected from the head plate to allow the fermenter to be autoclaved. In early fermenter models, the stirring shaft was connected through the head plate by replaceable rubber/silicone seals, which were vulnerable to damage and provided entry points of contamination. Later models have sealed units which are far more reliable.

Typically, maximum stirring rates of 100–150 rpm are used for cells in suspension, although this should be even lower (~40 rpm) for microcarrier cultures (see Chapter 10). Microcarriers are small spherical beads (diam. 200 µm) which can be suspended in a culture. Anchorage-dependent cells will attach and grow on the microcarrier surface.

In order to ensure adequate mixing at low stirring speeds, the culture vessels are designed with a round bottom, which distinguishes them from the flat-bottomed bacterial fermenters. Impeller blades which are fitted at the end of mechanical drive shafts are designed to allow vertical as well as horizontal liquid flow. The pitched-blade or marine type impellers are particularly suitable (*Figure 9.5*).

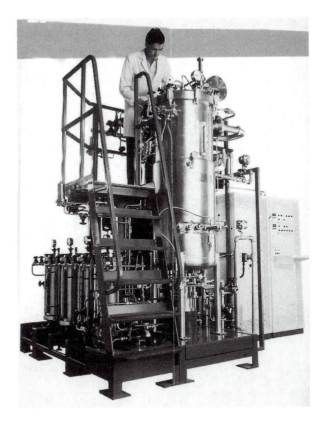

Figure 9.4

Stirred tank bioreactor for animal cells (500 liter).

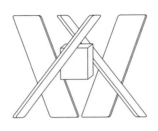

Pitched

Marine

Figure 9.5

External motor driven impellers.

2.2   Temperature control

High-power element heaters used in bacterial fermenters are avoided in mammalian cell cultures. At low agitation speeds the heat dissipation from such elements is insufficient to prevent localized heating in the culture. The temperature is usually controlled by a thermocirculator which pumps heated water (normally at 37°C) around an outer jacket or, for larger fermenters, through coiled pipes within the culture. An alternative system involves circulating warm air through an open-ended fermenter jacket. For low-volume bioreactors, external heating pads can be used to maintain the temperature.

2.3   pH control

The optimal pH for animal cell cultures is around pH 7.4 and maximum cell growth occurs if this is maintained. However, without buffering or external control this pH could fluctuate during culture and may decrease to a level that would eventually inhibit growth.

An enriched CO_2 atmosphere as provided by an incubator can decrease these fluctuations (see Chapter 3). Here, pH is controlled by gassing the cultures with CO_2. However, this buffering capacity is limited and would be inadequate for the high cell densities that can normally be expected in well-controlled fermenters. Further pH control by gaseous CO_2 is limited by the available head space in some industrial bioreactors. Typically a 1-liter culture at 2×10^6 cells/ml requires a gas flow of 100 ml/min into a head space with a 1-liter capacity.

An alternative method of pH control is by direct acid or alkali addition from a peristaltic pump. Normally during growth only alkali addition is required to offset the net acidic production from cellular metabolism. Low-volume addition of a concentrated sodium bicarbonate is often used in preference to sodium hydroxide because of the danger of over-shooting the set-point with the stronger alkali. These additions are normally governed by a computer-controlled pump or gas valve to a pre-set pH value (see Section 3). Acid (e.g. HCl) may also be added from an external source. However, this is usually not required as lactic acid is normally produced by cell metabolism and causes the culture pH to decrease during growth.

A typical set-up for CO_2 control of culture pH in a bioreactor is shown in *Figure 9.6*. The rotameters indicate the rate of gas flow into the culture, which can be controlled by the flow regulators. The electronic pH controller regulates the on/off function of the control valve.

2.4   Oxygen supply

The supply of oxygen to satisfy cell metabolism is one of the major problems associated with culture scale-up. The oxygen consumption rate of mammalian cells varies from 0.06–0.6 mmol/liter/hour for a culture at 10^6 cells/ml. In small cultures (T-flasks, etc.), this oxygen demand can be satisfied by gas diffusion from the head space through the culture surface. However, with increasing culture volume, the surface–volume ratio decreases. At cultures of 1 liter and above, the surface–volume ratio is generally too low to satisfy the overall oxygen demand at this cell concentration.

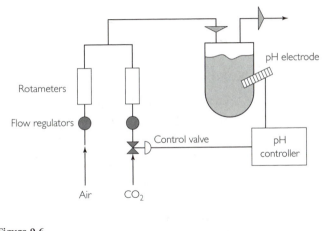

Figure 9.6

CO_2 control of culture pH in a bioreactor (from Kilburn, 1991).

The surface–volume ratio of a bioreactor is normally defined by the aspect ratio. For a cylindrical-shaped bioreactor, the aspect ratio = diameter/ height of culture (*Figure 9.7*).

If the cells utilize oxygen faster than it can be supplied, then the dissolved oxygen concentration of the culture media decreases eventually to a level that does not support cell growth. Thus, to avoid oxygen depletion, the oxygen transfer rate (OTR) across the liquid surface must be increased above the oxygen utilization rate (OUR) of the cells. In a simple fermenter containing 10^6 cells/ml and with an aspect ratio of one, oxygen supplied by diffusion will become limiting at around 1 liter. This is the critical volume at which OTR = OUR.

To satisfy the OUR at higher culture volumes, a continuous supply of oxygen is required. The following points must also be considered in developing a system for oxygen supply:

■ the solubility of oxygen in an air-saturated aqueous solution is low (0.22 mM at 37°C). This is the maximum concentration of oxygen in

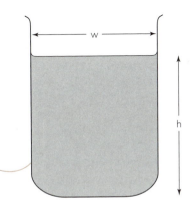

Figure 9.7

Aspect ratio = width/height of culture.

culture media which is in equilibrium with air and is referred to as '100% air saturation';

■   growth of many animal cell lines has been found to be optimal at a dissolved oxygen level below the maximum oxygen solubility and corresponding to 20–50% of air saturation.

Control of the oxygen supply

The dissolved oxygen level of a culture can be monitored by a sterilizable oxygen probe (*Figure 9.8*). This is fitted with a gas-permeable membrane to allow oxygen into an electrolyte contained in an inner chamber. The resulting reaction produces an electrical response that can be measured from a calibration based on differences between nitrogen-gassed (0%) and air-saturated water (100%).

The dissolved oxygen can be controlled by the opening of a valve when the value decreases below a predetermined set-point. Some of the strategies for control are shown in *Figure 9.9*. The action may increase the air flow in an airlift bioreactor (a), increase sparged oxygen in a stirred tank bioreactor (b), control the relative distribution of a combination of gases flowing into an airlift bioreactor (c) or sparge into a cell-free protected space of the bioreactor (d).

Oxygen vs air

The OTR can be increased by filling the head space with oxygen instead of air. This increases the OTR by a factor of about five and increases the critical volume or cell density at which OUR = OTR. Air contains oxygen at ~21%. Therefore, the partial pressure of oxygen in air is 1/5th of that in pure oxygen.

Oxygen solubility in culture media can also be increased (up to ×20) by the addition of some liquid perfluorocarbons (Riess and LeBlanc, 1982).

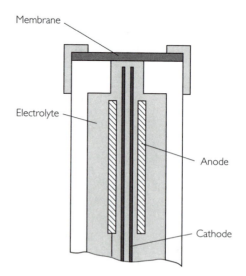

Figure 9.8

Membrane-covered oxygen electrode.

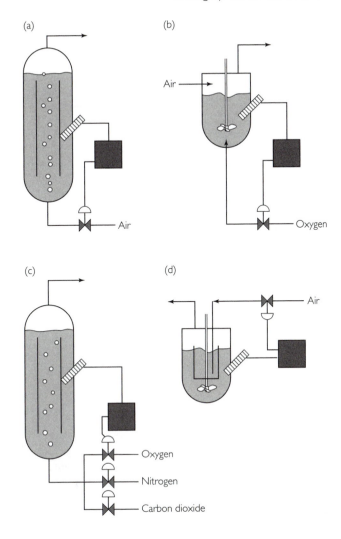

Figure 9.9

Strategies for controlling dissolved oxygen (from Kilburn, 1991).

However, both these options are expensive and do not allow indefinite scale-up possibilities.

Sparging

Direct aeration by sparging is commonly performed in bacterial cultures and is by far the simplest operation for supplying oxygen. However, cell damage can be caused by this process. This damage is associated with gas bubbles bursting at the culture surface. Cells may attach to the bubbles as they are formed in the sparger and can be carried to the liquid surface where bubble bursting can cause a significant shear force to damage the cells (*Figure 9.10*). A further problem is that sparging through the high protein content of mammalian culture media can cause excessive foaming, particularly in serum-supplemented media. Serum-free media with a low protein content are less

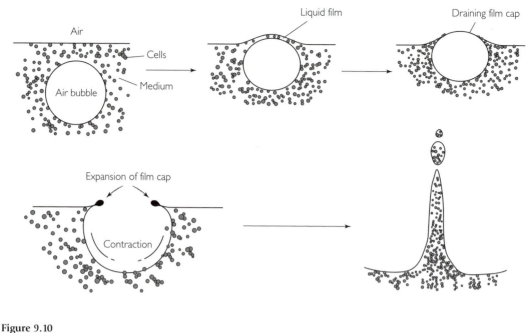

Figure 9.10

Bubble bursting causes cell death on the liquid surface.

susceptible to foaming, although the cells are less well protected against damage associated with agitation. Intermittent (rather than continuous) sparging can reduce damage to cells.

Chemical protective agents can be used to reduce cell damage and foam formation and these may be added to cultures that may be susceptible to such problems. These are mainly synthetic polymers and include Pluronic (a mixed glycol polymer), polyvinyl alcohol (PVA) and polyvinyl pyrrolidone (PVP). These reagents can be useful in culture but some of them may be difficult to remove during subsequent product purification (see Chapter 11).

An alternative method of reducing foam and bubble damage is to surround the gas sparger by a fine-mesh cage which can isolate the aeration process from the main cell population. This prevents the formation of bubbles in the culture. This is the basis of the Celligen unit – a bench-top fermenter designed by New Brunswick.

Indirect aeration

Indirect aeration of cultures can involve medium sparging in a secondary vessel. Such external oxygenation can alleviate the problems of air bubble or foam damage to cells and is particularly suitable for bioreactor configurations that involve media recirculation.

Diffusion via tubing

Oxygen can be supplied by gas diffusion through thin-walled silicone tubing. The tubing is submerged in the liquid medium and is supplied with air or oxygen under pressure. This system requires long lengths of tubing – at least

1 meter per 2 liters of culture. This may be unwieldy but can be overcome by adequate twining or binding of the tubing. Such a system is available in fermenters designed by Applikon and Braun.

3.   Process control

Maximum productivity and consistency between runs can be maintained if critical culture parameters are controlled and maintained at their optimal values (Kilburn, 1991). This is helped by using sterilizable probes connected to computer control systems. A number of culture parameters, including temperature, pH, oxygen, and foam level, can be controlled by this method. The output from each probe is transmitted electronically to a control unit where the value is compared to a predetermined set-point.

A deviation of the probe output from the set-point activates a corrective measure to shift the culture parameter towards the optimal conditions. This involves the activation of a pump to feed alkali, anti-foam, or oxygen into the culture or switch on a heating system. A modulated feedback controller is commonly used in fermenter systems (*Figure 9.11*). This is an electronic control system that ensures against large fluctuations around the set-point. A well-designed feedback system can reduce these oscillations and maintain the parameters very close to the set-point throughout the culture period. This avoids the type of changes that occur in small-volume cultures in the laboratory.

A modulated feedback controller of any of these culture parameters operates by proportional/integral/derivative (PID) control. This has three features of modulation which may be adjusted by proportional control, integral control or derivative time.

Proportional control

The output of the controller is proportional to the error signal.

$$\theta = \theta_0 + k.E$$

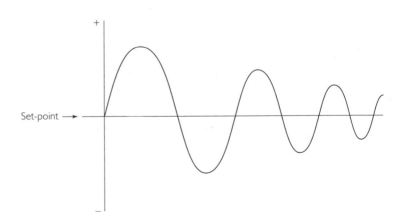

Figure 9.11

Modulated feedback control.

where θ = output signal of the controller, θ_0 = output signal when the error is zero, k = controller gain or proportional band, and E = error or deviation from the set-point.

Integral control

The output of the controller is a function of the integral of error and time. Here, the control action increases with time as long as the error is registered.

$$\theta = \theta_0 + \frac{1}{t_I} \cdot \int E.dt$$

where t_I = integral time constant.

Derivative time

The output of the controller is a function of the rate of change of the error.

$$\theta = \theta_0 + t_d \cdot \frac{dE}{dt}$$

where t_d = derivative time constant.

PID combines these three features. The values of the proportional band, integral time constant and derivative time constant may be adjusted on some controllers so as to optimize control of the culture parameters in a bioreactor.

The limitation to further development of these control systems is the availability of suitable probes for continuous measurement. Reliable, sterilizable probes for pH, oxygen and temperature control are presently available for cell cultures. It would undoubtedly be advantageous to control other critical factors such as nutrient concentrations by feeding from pumps. This would allow nutrients such as glucose and amino acids to be maintained at their optimal concentrations in culture. Such an optimal environment for cell growth and metabolism could limit the accumulation of adverse metabolic products such as lactic acid and ammonia. pH decreases with lactic acid formation. Ammonia inhibits cell growth.

Glucose and biomass probes are available but up to now have not been considered sufficiently reliable or cost-effective for continuous, routine use in animal cell fermenters.

4.   Alternative types of bioreactors

Although the STR is the most widely used type of bioreactor for large-scale cell cultures, and certainly the type recommended for laboratory work (up to 5 liters), there are a number of alternative systems that have been developed for culture scale-up.

4.1   Airlift fermenter

This type of fermenter consists of a tall column with an inner draught tube (Wood and Thompson, 1987) (*Figure 9.12*). Fluid circulation is provided by a stream of air which passes through the inside of the draught tube. This is a simple system without mechanical components and therefore not susceptible to breakdown. Bubble or foam damage is minimized by having a long

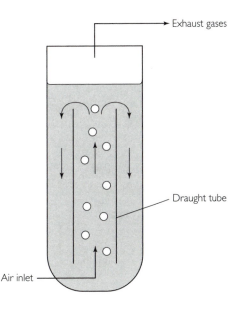

Exhaust gases

Draught tube

Air inlet

Figure 9.12

Airlift fermenter.

column, since it has been shown that maximum cell damage occurs at the point of bubble bursting at the top of the liquid column. An airlift fermenter (>1000 liters) has been used routinely for the production of bulk quantities of monoclonal antibodies from hybridomas by Lonza/Celltech in the UK.

4.2 Hollow-fiber bioreactor

This consists of bundles of synthetic, semipermeable hollow fibers, which offer a matrix for cell growth similar to the vascular system *in vivo* (Tyo *et al.*, 1988). The bioreactor is based on equipment originally developed for hemodialysis with a cartridge containing several thousand minute capillary-like plastic tubules (fibers) with perfusable membrane walls (*Figure 9.13*). Liquid can flow through the fibers (the intracapillary space) or through the space between the fibers (the extracapillary space). In the normal operation culture medium is pumped through the intracapillary space and a hydrostatic pressure permits the exchange of nutrients and waste products across the capillary wall. The cells and large-molecular-weight products are held in the extracapillary space. They grow to very high densities equivalent to the characteristics of tissue (up to 10^9 cells/ml) as could be seen from micrographs of a cross-section of several fibers. Medium is pumped into the fibers creating a relatively high pressure within the intracapillary space forcing nutrients through the pores into the extracapillary space. The perfusion of the medium provides efficient exchange of nutrients, gases and metabolites. The molecular weight cut-off of the fiber is normally 6000–10 000 Da.

A major limitation of this type of system is that the pressure difference that may be established along the length of fibers can cause nutrient gradients and uneven cell growth. Such pressure differences and gradients become an increasing problem with scale-up. The design of the 'Acusyst'

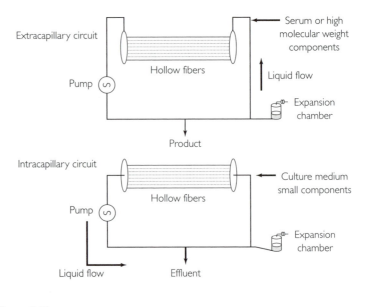

Figure 9.13

Hollow-fiber bioreactor.

hollow-fiber system was intended to correct this problem. Here the pressure differential between the intra- and extracapillary space is continuously monitored by sensors which serve to control the opening and closing of valves which in turn affect the capillary pressure.

The exchange of molecules through the fiber wall occurs in phases governed by a cyclic mode of pressure changes which prevent undue gradients developing along the fibers. This hollow-fiber system is suitable for both anchorage-dependent and -independent cells. Continuous operation allows a high rate of product recovery from a stationary high-density culture held in the extracapillary space over a long period of time. Hollow-fiber bioreactors can be operated continuously for several months.

4.3   Packed-bed or fixed-bed bioreactor

This type of bioreactor consists of a static support matrix for the attachment and growth of anchorage-dependent cells. Cell growth is supported by a continuous flow of medium. The design of these bioreactors attempts to maximize the surface area available for growth in a given volume. Three examples of bioreactors designed for such a purpose are given.

The glass bead column

The example shown in *Figure 9.14* consists of a bed of solid glass beads with a diameter of 3–5 mm (Whiteside and Spier, 1981). The glass beads offer a good surface for cell attachment. Cells are allowed to attach and grow on the bead surface. The medium is recirculated through the packed bed by a pump and oxygenated by an input of air in a secondary vessel. An attempt is made to ensure an even distribution of cells over the matrix so as to maximize yield and to prevent any concentration gradient of cells in the system.

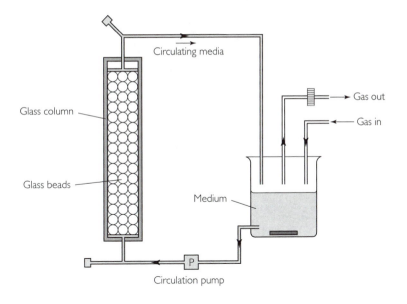

Circulating media

Gas out

Gas in

Glass column

Glass beads

Medium

P

Circulation pump

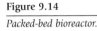

Figure 9.14

Packed-bed bioreactor.

In the column of glass beads this problem may be prevented by inoculating cells through a perforated tube, placed centrally through the vertical height of the column. Precoating the glass beads with fibronectin can ensure rapid cell attachment.

The ceramic bioreactor

Although now largely in disuse the commercially developed 'Opticell' system was an attempt to offer a large surface area in a series of multiple channels which run through the length of a ceramic cylinder (Lydersen, 1987). Each channel is a square with 1 mm sides and an inner surface area for cell attachment (*Figure 9.15*). A cartridge consists of a ceramic cylinder, which can vary in size, loaded into a glass surround through which the culture medium is pumped. A porous ceramic allows growth within the walls of the channels and is suitable for nonadherent cell lines whereas a nonporous smooth surface can allow the attachment and growth of anchorage-dependent cells. The basic ceramic cylinder is 30 cm in length with a radius of 4 cm and is supplied with a medium reservoir of up to 20 liters. Several cartridges can be operated in series to increase the scale of the process. The mode of operation of the Opticell ceramic system is by constant recirculation of medium through the channels of the cartridge. This allows the necessary distribution of nutrients and permits the re-oxygenation of the medium outside the culture. Extracellularly released products can be isolated from the spent medium which may be continuously siphoned into a harvest flask from the main reservoir at a preset rate. The main reservoir is replenished by fresh medium from a feed tank.

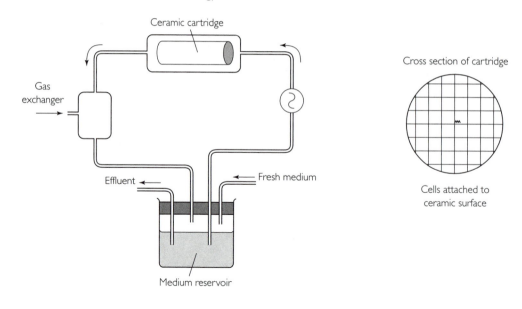

Cross section of cartridge

Cells attached to
ceramic surface

Figure 9.15

Opticell ceramic system.

The Cell Cube

A third example (the Cell Cube) is shown in *Figure 9.16*. This consists of a stack of 20 cm^2 polystyrene plates spaced 1 mm apart by rigid spacers and in a case that can be sterilized (Aunins *et al.*, 2003). The cells attach to either side of each polystyrene plate and are supported by the flow of culture medium between the plates. In the Cell Cube multiple inlet ports ensure the upward flow of liquid medium. Each port is shaped like a nozzle to ensure maximum distribution of the liquid over the plates. These design features ensure the even distribution of cells over the available surface (*Figure 9.17*).

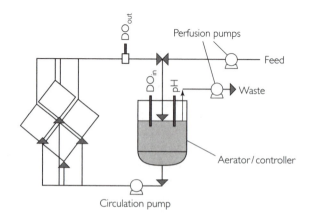

Figure 9.16

The Cell Cube bioreactor (from Aunins et al., 2003).

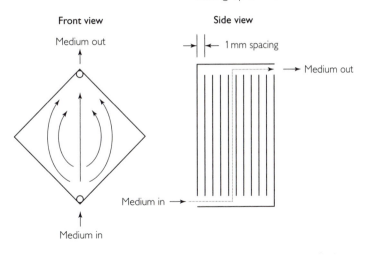

Figure 9.17

Fluid flow in the Cell Cube (from Aunis et al., *2003).*

Such packed-bed or fixed-bed bioreactors are suitable for scale-up and commercial production of vaccines from the viruses that can be propagated on the cells. A commonly used alternative for anchorage-dependent cell growth is the use of microcarriers which are small beads that can be suspended in culture and offer a surface for cell attachment. These are pseudo-suspension cultures and can be conducted in stirred tank bioreactors (see Chapter 10).

4.4   Fluidized-bed reactor

In this system, cells immobilized or entrapped in beads are held in suspension in a column by an upward flow of liquid medium that is recirculated by pumping (Runstadler and Cernek, 1988) (*Figure 9.19*). Some fluidized-bed reactors have been designed in a funnel shape with a fluid flow from the narrow bottom. The density and bead size are generally high so that a linear fluid velocity supports the beads in a relatively homogeneous suspension. This can be compared to the use of microcarriers in a stirred tank reactor (see Chapter 10). The bead characteristics need to be optimized to suit the bioreactor. Porous collagen and alginate beads have been used successfully. Bead densities can be increased as required by the addition of a heavy metal.

In the example shown (*Figure 9.18*) (the fluidized-bed bioreactor; the Cytopilot) the fluid circulation is integrated into a single module. The module consists of an upper and lower cylindrical chamber. The lower chamber consists of a magnetic stirrer, probes, a sample and heating jacket allowing the flow of temperature-controlled water. This is separated from the upper chamber by a porous distributor plate. The upper chamber is a tall column containing the porous microcarriers suspended in culture medium and into which the cells are entrapped. Liquid is allowed to circulate via a cell-free inner tube by a magnetically driven stirrer, which controls the degree of fluidization of the microcarriers (*Figure 9.19*). The microcarriers used

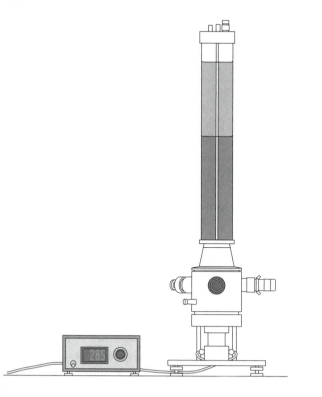

Figure 9.18

Cytopilot Mini.

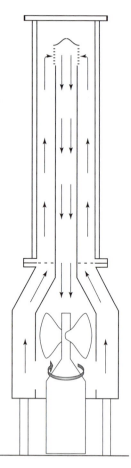

in this bioreactor are macroporous, allowing easy entry of the cells on inoculation and an inner capacity to allow growth to high cell densities. The microcarriers (Cytoline) are weighted to a density of around 1.3 g/cm^3 allowing high sedimentation rates in the fluidized column. The bioreactor is run in a perfusion mode, allowing a continuous flow of effluent containing the cell product. The culture is simultaneously provided with an equivalent flow of fresh medium to maintain a constant culture volume in the bioreactor.

References

Aunins, J.G., Bader, B., Caola, A. *et al.* (2003) Fluid mechanics, cell distribution and environment in Cell Cube bioreactors. *Biotechnol. Progress* **19**: 2–8.

Kilburn, D.G. (1991) Monitoring and control of bioreactors. In: Butler, M. (ed.) *Mammalian Cell Biotechnology: A Practical Approach*, pp.159–185. Oxford University Press, Oxford.

Lydersen, B.K. (1987) Perfusion cell culture system based on ceramic matrices. In: Lydersen, B.K. (ed.) *Large Scale Culture Technology*, pp. 169–192. J. Wiley, Chichester.

Riess, J.G. and LeBlanc, M. (1982) Solubility and transport phenomena in perfluorochemicals relevant to blood substitution and other biomedical applications. *Pure Appl. Chem.* **54**: 2383–2406.

Runstadler Jr., P.W. and Cernek, S.R. (1988) Large-scale fluidized-bed, immobilized cultivation of animal cells at high densities. In Spier, R.E. and Griffiths J.B. (eds) *Animal Cell Biotechnology*, Vol. 3, pp. 305–320. Academic Press, London.

Figure 9.19

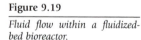

Fluid flow within a fluidized-bed bioreactor.

Tyo, M.A., Bulbulian, B.J., Menken, B.Z. and Murphy, T.J. (1988) Large-scale mammalian cell culture utilizing Acusyst technology. In: Spier, R.E. and Griffiths J.B. (eds) *Animal Cell Biotechnology*, Vol. 3, pp. 358–371. Academic Press, London.

Whiteside, J.P. and Spier, R.E. (1981) The scale-up from 0.1 to 100 litre of a unit process system based on 3 mm diameter glass spheres for the production of four strains of FMDV from BHK monolayer cells. *Biotechnol. Bioeng.* **23**: 551–565.

Wood, L.A. and Thompson, P.W. (1987) Applications of the air lift fermenter. *Appl. Biochem. Biotechnol.* **15**: 131–143.

Further reading

Bliem, R. and Katinger, H. (1988) Scale-up engineering in animal cell technology. *Trends Biotechnol.* **6**: 190–195.

Feder, J. and Tolbert, W.R. (eds) (1985) *Large Scale Mammalian Cell Culture*. Academic Press, New York.

Griffiths, B. (1986) Scaling-up of animal cell cultures. In: Freshney, R.I. (ed.) *Animal Cell Culture: A Practical Approach*, pp. 33–69. IRL Press at Oxford University Press, Oxford.

Handa-Corrigan, A. (1991) Bioreactors for mammalian cells. In: Butler, M. (ed.) *Mammalian Cell Biotechnology: A Practical Approach*, pp.139–158. Oxford University Press, Oxford.

Lubiniecki, A.S. (ed.) (1990) *Large-Scale Mammalian Cell Culture Technology*. Marcel Dekker, New York.

Lydersen, B.K. (ed.) (1987) *Large Scale Culture Technology*. Hanser, New York.

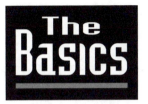

Chapter 10

Modes of culture for high cell densities

In this chapter the characteristics of simple batch cultures are compared to alternative modes of culture that allow continuous or semicontinuous feeding. These continuous culture systems are valuable for obtaining high cell yields even from low-volume cultures. This enables product yields to be increased by higher cell densities in culture without necessarily a scale-up in volume. This is called 'process intensification'. Cell immobilization into suitable inert carrier beads can help in obtaining these high yields, particularly for anchorage-dependent cells and is explained in this chapter.

1. Batch culture

In the previous chapter different bioreactor types were considered from the simple stirred tank reactors to the more complex packed-bed or hollow-fiber systems. These bioreactors can be classified in terms of their mixing characteristics as homogeneous or heterogeneous. In the stirred tank reactor, homogeneous mixing of all culture components is maintained. A cellular substrate introduced into the bioreactor will blend immediately into the culture and will gradually decrease in concentration as cells grow (*Figure 10.1*).

On the other hand, the packed-bed and hollow-fiber systems can be characterized as heterogeneous. A substrate introduced into the inlet will flow as a single band through the tubular bioreactor without back mixing. This is called 'plug-flow' (*Figure 10.2*).

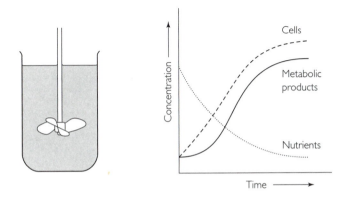

Figure 10.1

Kinetics of a batch culture.

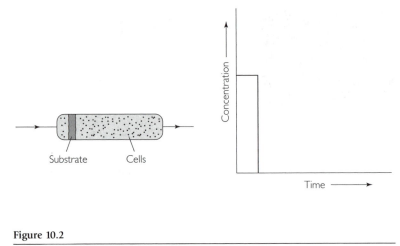

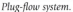

Substrate   Cells

Figure 10.2

Plug-flow system.

The graph shows the change in concentration of a substrate at the inlet of such a bioreactor. The concentration will decrease along the length of the bioreactor. For better utilization of substrates such heterogeneous systems are normally fitted with a loop so that the culture medium is continuously recycled over the growing cells. This is called a quasi-homogeneous system in which the concentration of any substrate will decrease in a series of steps (*Figure 10.3*). Here the kinetics of substrate utilization approximates what happens in a homogeneous culture.

All the above are examples of closed or batch cultures. The cells are inoculated and the culture is left for several days until the final density is reached. In a closed system nothing is added or removed during the culture, apart from small volume samples for analysis.

However, it is important to realize that the cells are exposed to a constantly changing environment of substrates that are removed from the

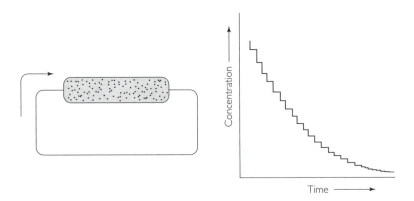

Figure 10.3

Medium recycled through the culture.

medium and products that are secreted from the cells. Any nutrient will gradually decrease from an initially high concentration to a low concentration following growth of the cells. These changes lead to a gradually deteriorating environment for cell growth, which is likely to cease at around 10^6 cells/ml because of one or more of the following factors:

- depletion of an essential nutrient;
- accumulation of an inhibitor;
- a complete cover of the available growth surface (for anchorage-dependent cells).

Media components are consumed by the cells at variable rates, glutamine and glucose being the substrates consumed most rapidly during growth. Their utilization leads to the gradual formation of ammonia and lactate as metabolic by-products. Substrate consumption or product formation is usually expressed as a specific rate as pmol/cell per hour or μmol/10^6 cells per hour. This measurement of specific substrate uptake (Q_S) or product formation (Q_P) is widely used in the analysis of media changes during batch culture.

$$Q_S = -\frac{dS}{dt} \cdot \frac{1}{N_v}$$

$$Q_P = \frac{dP}{dt} \cdot \frac{1}{N_v}$$

where dS/dt and dP/dt represent the rate of utilization of a substrate or rate of formation of a product, and N_v is the viable cell concentration. Of course, in a culture the value of N_v changes over time. During exponential growth this value can be derived from the equation:

$$Q_S = \frac{\Delta S}{T} \cdot \frac{\ln N - \ln N_0}{N - N_0}$$

where ΔS is the change in concentration of the substrate of the time period T, and N_0 and N are the initial and final cell concentrations, respectively.

This equation is applicable during the exponential growth phase only. However, over the whole culture where the growth goes through several phases, the equation becomes:

$$Q_S = \frac{\Delta S}{\int_0^t N_v \, dt}$$

The integral represents the area under the growth curve (N vs time) from time zero to each time point. If such a calculation is made for each time point a series of integral values is generated. If N represents viable cell concentrations then the integrals are often referred to as viability indices. The value of Q_S (or Q_P) can be determined from the slope of the plot of substrate (or product) concentration and the integral values. A single straight line indicates a constant rate of substrate uptake per cell throughout the culture. In some cases distinct phases of uptake or production rates may be observed. *Figure 10.4* shows typical data from a batch culture in which cells grow to a maximum density of 10^6 cells/ml, as a substrate at an initial concentration of 25 mM is utilized. Transformation of these data (*Figure 10.5*) suggests two

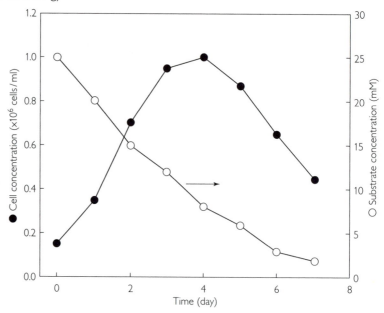

Figure 10.4

Cell growth and substrate concentration.

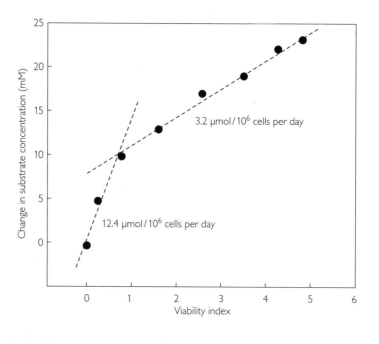

Figure 10.5

Viability index vs substrate utilization.

phases of uptake during culture with a high Q_S during the cell growth phase and a lower Q_S during the stationary and decline phases. The same type of plot can be used to determine production rates of metabolic by-products such as lactate and ammonia.

Another useful measure is the growth yield ($Y_{N,S}$) which is the measure of the number of cells generated following the consumption of a millimole of substrate.

$$Y = \frac{\Delta N}{\Delta S}$$

2. Fed-batch culture

The final cell yield attained in a batch culture may be dependent upon the concentration of available nutrients or the accumulation of metabolic by-products. When a situation is reached whereby a specific nutrient is limiting or a by-product becomes toxic then cell growth will stop. Attempts to increase the cell yield further will depend upon the nutrient supply or the removal of by-products. This will result in gradually higher cell yields as these limitations are overcome (*Figure 10.6*). If all these growth limitations are removed, the cell yield should reach concentrations found in tissue (*in vivo*). However, it is difficult to identify the sequential list of limiting parameters above densities of 10^7 cells/ml, as indicated by the question mark in *Figure 10.6*.

In an open system cells are supplied with nutrients during the course of culture in an attempt to increase the cell yield. The simplest system is the fed-batch culture which involves controlled nutrient feeding. This can involve partial media changes at regular intervals or it can involve the addition of specific nutrients at critical stages of the culture. It is useful to identify the limiting nutrients before setting up a fed-batch culture. This can lead to the addition of a concentrate of specific amino acids or glucose at daily intervals in an attempt to increase the final cell yield. However, despite such

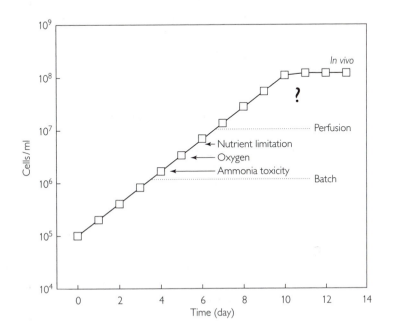

Figure 10.6

Limiting factors associated with cell growth.

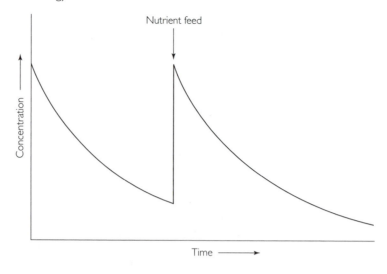

Figure 10.7

Kinetics of a fed-batch culture.

feeding, metabolic products will still accumulate eventually to growth-inhibitory concentrations. *Figure 10.7* indicates the changes in nutrient concentration during a fed-batch process.

3. Continuous culture

This term is applied to an open system with a continuous feed of medium and removal of 'spent' medium. Cell growth continues for longer periods in a continuous culture compared to a batch culture. There are two main types of continuous culture:

■ chemostat culture: where the cells are removed continuously from the fermenter;
■ perfusion culture: where the cells are retained in the fermenter.

3.1 Chemostat culture

In this system spent medium and cells are removed continuously through an outlet tube as in *Figure 10.8* (Tovey, 1985). The state of the culture is dependent upon the flow rate of fresh medium. This is expressed as a dilution rate (D) which is defined as the medium flow rate (F) divided by the culture volume (V):

$$D = \frac{F}{V}$$

The dilution rate of a chemostat culture of mammalian cells should normally be between 0.2–1.0 volume/day. This is the proportion of the cell culture volume that is replaced in 1 day. Another useful term is the residence time (= 1/D), which is the mean time that an added component remains in the culture.

A steady-state equilibrium is established when the cell growth rate equals the dilution rate. The units for specific growth rate and dilution rate are the

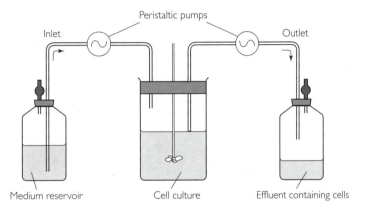

Figure 10.8

Continuous culture.

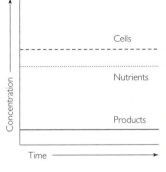

Figure 10.9

The kinetics of a chemostat culture.

same (e.g. 0.2 d^{-1} or 0.008 h^{-1}). At equilibrium the concentrations of cells, nutrients and products are constant as shown in *Figure 10.9*. If the dilution rate is changed then a new steady state will be established. If new components are added to the medium that is pumped into the bioreactor, a steady state will be re-established after 3–5 volume changes of the culture.

The chemostat is a self-regulating system in which a temporary decrease in cell concentration will cause a corresponding increase in growth rate, and an increase in cell concentration has the reverse effect. Thus, the steady-state conditions are always restored, although each new equilibrium will take 3–5 volume changes to be established.

In the chemostat the specific growth rate (μ) of the cell population is maintained at a level below a maximum value (μ_{max}) by the concentration of a limiting substrate (S). This is defined by the Monod equation:

$$\mu = \mu_{max} \cdot \frac{S}{K_s + S}$$

where S is the variable concentration of the limiting substrate, and K_s is a constant related to the affinity of the cell–substrate interaction.

When S is significantly higher than K_s then the nutrients are in excess and the growth rate is at the maximal value. As the substrate concentration declines to the value of K_s then so does the growth rate. The saturation constant (K_s) from the Monod equation represents the substrate concentration at which the specific growth rate is half the maximum rate ($\mu = \mu_{max}/2$). This parallels the relationship between substrates and enzymes as expressed in the well-known Michaelis-Menten equation (*Figure 10.10*).

In a continuous culture the growth rate will increase as the concentration of the limiting substrate is increased, until a critical value is reached when cell growth continues at its maximum rate. If the dilution rate is increased beyond this point, then the cells will be washed out of the culture. This occurs when the medium is pumped out of the culture faster than the cells can grow. Mammalian cells can be grown in a chemostat culture in which the glucose concentration is limiting, although in many cases the limiting substrate may be unknown.

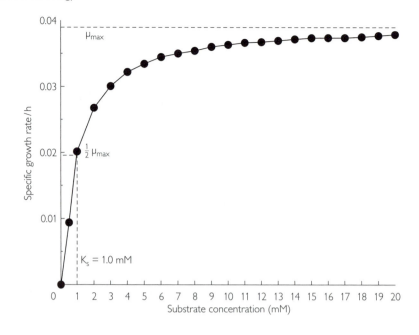

Figure 10.10

The effect of substrate concentration on specific growth rate.

The following are the kinetic equations that define a chemostat culture. The increase in cell number:

$$\frac{dN}{dt} = \mu.N - D.N$$

where $\mu.N$ represents an increase in cell number from growth and $D.N$ represents a decrease in cell number from the effluent of the culture.

If the specific growth rate is greater than the dilution rate ($\mu > D$) then dN/dt is positive and the concentration of cells in the culture will increase.

If the specific growth rate is lower than the dilution rate ($\mu < D$) then dN/dt is negative and the concentration of cells in the culture will decrease. If this is maintained then the cell number will eventually decrease to zero indicating complete wash-out from the culture.

At steady state:

$$\frac{dN}{dt} = 0$$

at which $\mu = D$.

This is true so long as D is below the critical dilution rate at which cell wash-out occurs. It is important to know what values of D make a steady state possible. This may be determined from knowledge of the yield coefficient:

Yield coefficient, Y = number of cells formed/moles of substrate utilized

This can be expressed as:

$$\frac{dN}{dt} = Y \cdot \frac{dS}{dt}$$

The rate of change of substrate concentration in a chemostat can be equated to the rate of input minus the output in the effluent and minus the cellular consumption. Thus:

$$\frac{dS}{dt} = D.S_R - D.S - \frac{\mu N}{Y}$$

where S_R is the substrate concentration in the input medium and S is the concentration in the culture or the effluent.

By combining the two equations above:

$$\frac{dN}{dt} = N\left(\mu_{max} \cdot \frac{S}{K_S + S} - D\right)$$

and

$$\frac{dS}{dt} = D.(S_R - S) - \mu_{max} \cdot \frac{S}{K_S + S} \cdot \frac{N}{Y}$$

If S_R and D are held constant and D does not exceed a critical value, then there are unique values of N and S for which both $dN/dt = 0$ and $dS/dt = 0$. These are the steady-state values of the cell concentration (N') and substrate concentration in the bioreactor (S'):

$$S' = K_S \cdot \left(\frac{D}{\mu_{max} - D}\right)$$

$$N' = Y.(S_R - S) = Y.\left(S_R - K_S \cdot \frac{D}{\mu_{max} - D}\right)$$

Over most of the range of possible dilution rate values, the steady-state concentration of the limiting substrate is very low. This indicates that it is almost completely consumed by the cells.

When D approaches the critical dilution rate (D_c) at which wash-out occurs, then unused substrate appears in the culture.

At D_c the substrate approaches the maximum value ($S = S_R$). Therefore

$$D_c = \mu_{max} \cdot \frac{S_R}{K_S + S_R}$$

Figure 10.11 shows the change in these parameters with a change in dilution rate.

The cell and product output from the chemostat increases with $D \times N$, which is the dilution rate times the cell concentration.

At D_c there is complete wash-out of cells. However at a lower value than this ($= D_m$) the maximum cellular output and production occurs. This value corresponds to the maximum growth rate (μ_{max}) of the cells.

3.2 Perfusion

An alternative type of open system involves medium perfusion (Griffiths, 1990). Here, the medium is pumped continuously through the culture, but the cells are retained in the bioreactor. This type of process is becoming increasingly popular for large-scale production (Tolbert *et al.*, 1988). The continuous supply of nutrients and removal of waste products promotes cell

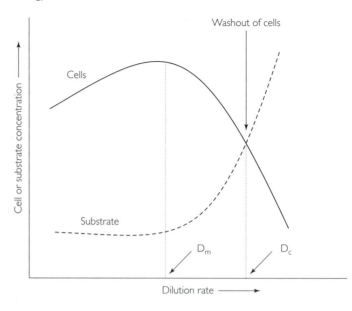

Figure 10.11

The effect of dilution rate on cell and substrate concentrations in a chemostat.

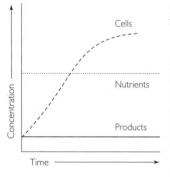

Figure 10.12

The kinetics of a perfusion culture.

growth to a greater extent than in a batch culture and allows a high cell density to be attained. Typically, final cell densities of $>10^7$ cells/ml will occur although this is dependent upon the perfusion rate. *Figure 10.12* shows the ideal kinetics of a perfusion culture with the nutrients maintained at a high concentration and the metabolic product concentration reduced to a minimum.

The advantages of the perfusion mode include high productivity from a high cell density and a low residence time of the product in the culture environment. The low residence time of a recombinant protein has the advantage of reduced risk from any protease and sialidase activity that may be released by the cells.

Cell separators

In a perfusion system, some device is required to separate the cells from the medium that is pumped out from the culture.

Open tube/gravitational settling

Gravitational separation depends upon a density difference between the particle and the surrounding liquid. This type of device is particularly well suited for microcarrier cultures, in which the cell-loaded microcarriers are heavy and sediment from an effluent column allowing a clear cell-free liquid to be withdrawn from the culture. A wide-bore tube positioned at the liquid surface of a culture creates a column of unstirred liquid in which the microcarriers can sediment. The small settling (or decanting) column is often sufficient to allow beads to gravitate back into the culture, enabling the medium to be pumped out (*Figure 10.13*). Cells immobilized in beads can be separated easily from the surrounding medium. The liquid column is

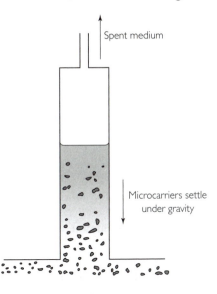

Figure 10.13

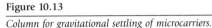

Column for gravitational settling of microcarriers.

maintained by a peristaltic pump. A column constructed from glass allows the separation to be seen (*Figure 10.14*). It is possible to maintain cell concentrations up to 10^7 cells/ml with such a system. Higher cell densities would require higher flow rates but this may lead to less efficient separation and the unwanted removal of cells from the bioreactor.

Unfortunately, this type of column separator will not operate efficiently for a suspension culture because the density of cells is not sufficiently different from the surrounding medium to allow separation. However, the

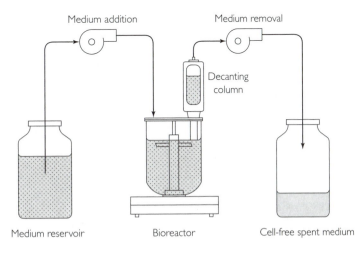

Figure 10.14

Continuous culture with a decanting column.

principle of gravitational separation can be applied in a lamella settler, in which the cells are separated in a series of closely packed parallel plates, normally inclined at a 45° angle. The key to this device is the large area offered for separation which allows cells to move down the lower surface of the separation space. Separation is aided by coating the plates with a material to prevent cell adhesion and also by continuous vibration.

Spin filter

This device involves a rotating mesh cage to allow medium flow but prevent cell wash-out (Thayer, 1973) (*Figure 10.15*). The cell-free effluent is withdrawn from within the filter. Rotation of the filter is required to prevent clogging. The device may be constructed from stainless steel with a variable mesh size. A mesh size of 5–15 microns is suitable for cell separation from a suspension culture whereas a higher mesh size of 70–150 microns is more suitable for a microcarrier culture. The major problem of the spin filter is the potential for fouling and blockage with cells over an extended period of use. Fouling of the spin filter causes a decrease in the effluent flow rate from the bioreactor. A high cell density contributes to fouling of the screen, although this problem can be eased by increasing the filter surface area or by using a high enough rotational velocity. Also, a higher mesh size could alleviate fouling but at the expense of a reduced efficiency of cell separation. It is possible to mount the stirring impeller and the spin filter on the same shaft. However, for large-scale bioreactors there is greater operational flexibility if the rotation of the two devices is controlled separately.

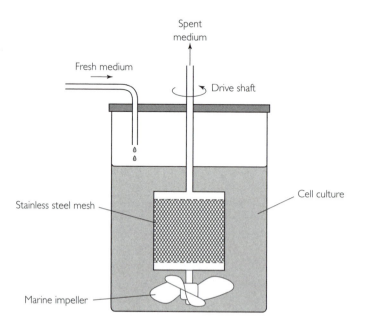

Figure 10.15

Spin filter.

Acoustic cell filtration

In this device the effluent from a culture is withdrawn through a resonator chamber, in which the liquid is subjected to an ultrasonic acoustic field at a frequency of about 2 MHz. A typical configuration of this system is provided by Applikon with their Biosep device. The standing sound wave, which is perpendicular to the outward flow of liquid, causes cells to aggregate and sediment back into the bioreactor. In its simplest operation, the perfusion pump runs continuously. However, there are some operational refinements that may improve the performance and efficiency of separation. One method is to operate the perfusion pump in a discontinuous cycle, which can incorporate a pause allowing cells to sediment. A typical cycle consists of a 20-second forward operation followed by a 6-second pause, in which the perfusion pump and acoustic field are switched off. Another refinement of the system is the incorporation of an external loop pump which flushes trapped cells back into the bioreactor against the main effluent flow.

Tangential flow filtration/loop reactor

The principle of this separation is that the culture is fed through hollow fibers, the walls of which are permeable. In this loop bioreactor the effluent from the stirred tank is pumped continuously through an external tangential flow filtration unit. A small ultrafiltration unit can separate cells from medium in the hollow fibers. The cells are returned to the stirred tank. The flow rate through the filtration unit is limited by high shear rates that can damage the cells. Membrane blockage can be a problem but is preventable by periodic back flushing and coating the inner surface with polyethylene glycol that prevents the build-up of protein. To scale-up the separation, a large number of short filtration units should be used in parallel.

4. Cell immobilization

The immobilization of cells on or inside particles suspended in culture medium offers an alternative mode of culture (Nilsson, 1987). Immobilization can involve the attachment of cells to a solid surface – which is the only way anchorage-dependent cells can grow. Alternatively, it can mean the entrapment of cells in small beads. In this section we will look at the properties of various immobilization systems. These immobilized systems are ideal for use with perfusion cultures.

4.1 Microcarriers for anchorage-dependent cells

At the laboratory scale, anchorage-dependent cells can be grown in Petri dishes, T-flasks or roller bottles (Chapter 3). However, these are limited in terms of the available surface area for growth. In order to increase cell yield or to design a process for large-scale production involving anchorage-dependent cells, a system offering a high growth surface to volume ratio is required.

Microcarrier cultures are designed to provide a pseudo-suspension culture for anchorage-dependent cells (Butler, 1987). Microcarriers are microscopic particles (normally with a diameter of about 200 μm) that are easily maintained in suspension in liquid medium (*Figure 10.16*). The suspension of microcarriers is maintained in a spinner flask which contains a

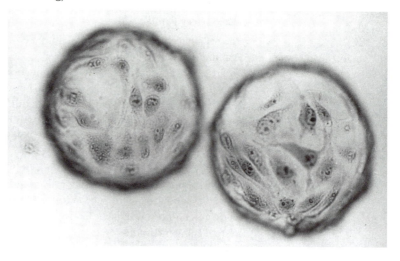

Figure 10.16

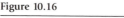

A confluent layer of BHK cells covers two microcarriers.

magnetic flea and a paddle suspended from a stirring shaft. The flask can be 100–500 ml in volume and should be placed on a specialized microcarrier stirring platform to allow a relatively slow and controlled stirring speed of around 40 rpm. These cultures are also suitable for scale-up and can be operated in simple stirred tanks in production processes (Protocol 10.1).

The major characteristics required of microcarriers are as follows:

■   small, to maximize the available surface area for cell growth;
■   light, to allow easy suspension in culture medium;
■   transparent, to allow easy observation of cell attachment and growth;
■   charged, to allow cell attachment onto the surface.

Microcarriers have been made from various materials including dextran, collagen and plastic. The surface is charged so as to ensure cell attachment. The density of the electrostatic charge on the microcarrier surface is critical to allow cell attachment and growth. The cells will then grow over the outer surface area until a monolayer is formed. Each microcarrier will accommodate 100–200 cells. It is important at inoculation that there is an even distribution of cells on the available microcarriers so that there are no 'empty' microcarriers at the end of the growth period. Also, it is important to ensure a stirring rate that allows the microcarriers to be suspended in the culture medium but does not cause damage to the cells. Cells can be detached from microcarriers by proteolytic enzymes (e.g. trypsin or collagenase) although, for processes that are designed for the production of a secreted cell product, cell removal may be unnecessary.

The advantages of microcarrier cultures

The potential of microcarriers for supporting cell growth can be realized from a calculation of the available surface area compared to that of a traditional system, the Roux bottle. A standard-sized Roux bottle has a surface area of 0.02 m^2 and can accommodate approximately 10^8 cells. In comparison 1 g (dry weight) of solid microcarriers (Cytodex) in 1 liter of culture provides a total surface area of 0.64 m^2 and can support 2×10^9 cells (equivalent to 20 Roux bottles). The handling operations involved in a 1-liter microcarrier culture are considerably simpler than those of 20 Roux bottle cultures, yet an equivalent cell yield is obtained. This comparison between a unit culture system (microcarrier) and a multiple culture system (Roux bottles) is illustrated in *Figure 10.17*. The advantages of a unit system become even clearer as the culture is scaled up to higher volume.

A key factor in obtaining a high cell yield in a microcarrier culture is to ensure that each bead accepts a viable cell at inoculation. This ensures full colonization of the available surface and limits the number of unoccupied beads at the end of the culture. Attachment of cells to beads has been shown to follow a Poisson distribution:

$$P = e^{-\lambda} \cdot \frac{\lambda^n}{n!}$$

where P = probability of a specific number (n) of cell hits per bead, and λ = ratio of cells to beads in culture at inoculation.

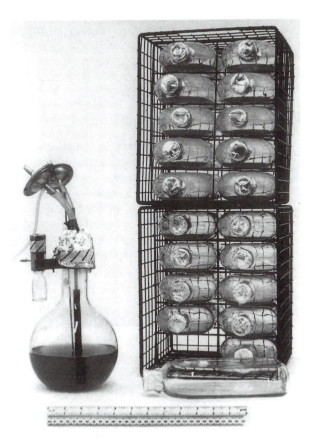

Figure 10.17

Comparison of a unit system and a multiple system.

The most useful result obtained from such an analysis is that a critical cell-to-bead inoculation ratio is necessary to ensure a negligible proportion of unoccupied microcarriers at the end of the culture. For most viable cell lines this critical ratio is >7. This ensures that the proportion of unoccupied microcarriers is <5% and the use of the available surface area is maximized.

A typical microcarrier culture is established with 1–3 g (dry weight) of microcarriers per liter. This allows a final cell density of around 2×10^6 cells/ml to be obtained from an inoculum density of 2×10^5 cells/ml. Higher microcarrier concentrations can be used (10–15 g/liter) but the disadvantages are the increasing difficulty of adequate culture agitation and the high cell inoculum densities required to enable correspondingly high yields.

Porous microcarriers

The original dextran microcarriers (e.g. Cytodex) are microporous. The pore size is not sufficient to allow cells to colonize the interior of the beads. However, macroporous carriers such as Cultispher are spherical gelatin microcarriers containing open channels large enough for cells to enter and continue growing within each bead. These have the advantage of increased surface area for cell attachment and an interior environment that may protect cells against adverse shear forces. Cells can attach to the beads or they may become trapped within the channels of the bead. This allows much higher cell–bead ratios than with solid microcarriers.

Porous microcarriers have been designed with various sizes and weights and are suitable for use in stirred tank or fluidized bed bioreactors (see Chapter 9). Some porous microcarriers have the capacity to accommodate up to 2000 cells per bead.

Choice of microcarriers

There is a wide selection of commercially available microcarrier types which differ in terms of the basic supporting matrix and the surface-coating material. The choice of microcarrier will depend upon the cell line used and the purpose or objectives of the culture. The most commonly used for surface attachment are Cytodex 1, 2 and 3. The Cytodex 1 is a cross-linked dextran matrix with positively charged N,N-diethylaminoethyl (DEAE) groups throughout the matrix. This type of microcarrier is suitable for the culture of a range of anchorage-dependent cells and is the most widely used. For relatively robust established cell lines, the charged-dextran microcarriers (such as Cytodex 1) have proved efficient and reliable. Cytodex 2 has a surface charge only and may reduce potential binding of cell products. Cytodex 3 has a collagen layer coupled to the surface and may enhance initial attachment of some cells, particularly those from primary tissue. Cultispher G is a macroporous gelatin and allows the cells to colonize the interior allowing higher cell numbers per bead. Under a microscope, the cells can easily be seen on the microcarrier surface. Staining with crystal violet is particularly useful as this highlights the nuclei against the transparent background of the microcarrier surface. Dextran-based microcarriers have been used extensively for the large-scale production of biologicals such as vaccines that are produced from anchorage-dependent cell lines.

Bead-to-bead transfer is an important operation for the scale-up of microcarrier cultures. This occurs by the addition of new microcarriers into an existing culture in which cells begin to colonize the new microcarriers. For this to occur efficiently, cells must detach from a confluent microcarrier surface and this will depend upon how firmly the cells are bound to the surface. For some cell lines this can occur in a low calcium medium or by a change of pH. For other cases a cocktail of trypsin and EDTA may be required.

If it is necessary to isolate high cell yields of fragile cell lines then microcarriers other than charged-dextran may be considered. Glass-coated or collagen-coated microcarriers are particularly suitable because detachment can be achieved efficiently and without significant cell damage by either trypsin or collagenase treatment. Detached cells can then be separated from microcarriers by sieving through a nylon mesh of appropriate size.

Gelatin-based or collagen-coated microcarriers may be a particularly good choice for the culture of primary cells. Such cells have fastidious growth requirements and attachment to a natural extracellular matrix may be advantageous. Microcarriers composed entirely of gelatin can be completely dissolved by proteolytic enzymes leaving the cells in suspension.

4.2 Immobilization of nonanchorage-dependent cells

The immobilization of nonanchorage-dependent cells into small beads can have many advantages such as:

■ protection against mechanical stress;
■ ease of continuous operation;
■ isolation of products.

Two systems have been found applicable:

■ encapsulation;
■ entrapment.

Cell entrapment

This can be accomplished in a variety of large polymers. Some of these are polysaccharides, with agarose being particularly well suited. The entrapment process involves mixing and agitating a suspension of cells in warm agarose with a hydrophobic liquid such as paraffin oil at a lower temperature. This causes the formation of small solid beads of agarose (100–200 μm) containing the suspended cells. The mechanical strength of the beads can be varied by using different agarose concentrations from 0.5 to 5%. Agarose is highly porous and will allow the free diffusion of high-molecular-weight substances through the matrix.

Growth of the entrapped cells in the beads can continue to high densities in bioreactors with high stirring speeds and rates of aeration. At high densities, some cell leakage can occur from the beads, but this may be prevented by careful growth control. Secreted cellular products accumulate in the medium which can then be easily separated from the entrapped cells – the system being ideally suited for continuous perfusion.

Encapsulation

Encapsulation is a modification of cell entrapment with cells enclosed in a semipermeable membrane which retains the cells and large secreted

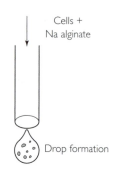

Cells +
Na alginate

Drop formation

CaCl$_2$ solution

Figure 10.18

Cell encapsulation.

molecules but allows the free diffusion of small molecules (Tyler, 1990). Spherical solid beads of calcium alginate can be formed by allowing a suspension of cells in sodium alginate to drip into a calcium chloride solution (*Figure 10.18*). An outer semipermeable membrane can be created by the addition of a basic polymer (e.g. polylysine) and the calcium alginate interior of the bead can then be re-liquefied by treatment with sodium citrate. The encapsulated cells are well protected against mechanical forces and can accumulate to high densities within the membrane. High-molecular-weight products are also retained within the membrane. This idea has been applied commercially to the growth of hybridomas. The secreted monoclonal antibodies accumulate to a high concentration within the bead matrix. Extraction of Mabs from beads of encapsulated cells is relatively easy because of the high concentration.

References

Butler, M. (1987) Growth limitations in microcarrier cultures. *Adv. Biochem. Eng. Biotechnol.* **34**: 57–84.

Griffiths, B. (1990) Perfusion systems for cell cultivation. In: Lubiniecki, A.S. (ed.) *Large-Scale Mammalian Cell Culture Technology*, pp. 217–250. Marcel Dekker, New York.

Nilsson, K. (1987) Methods for immobilizing animal cells. *Trends Biotechnol.* **5**: 73–78.

Thayer, P.S. (1973) Spin filter device for suspension cultures. In: Kruse P.F. Jr. and Patterson, M.K. (eds) *Tissue Culture: Methods and Applications*, pp. 345–351. Academic Press, New York.

Tolbert, W.R., Srigley, W.R. and Prior, C.P. (1988) Perfusion culture systems for large-scale pharmaceutical production. In: Spier, R.E. and Griffiths J.B. (eds) *Animal Cell Biotechnology*, Vol. 3, pp. 373–393. Academic Press, London.

Tovey, M.G. (1985) The cultivation of animal cells in continuous-flow culture. In: Spier, R.E. and Griffiths, J.B. (eds) *Animal Cell Biotechnology*, Vol. 1, pp.195–210. Academic Press, London.

Tyler, J.E. (1990) Microencapsulation of mammalian cells. In: Lubiniecki, A.S. (ed.) *Large-Scale Mammalian Cell Culture Technology*, pp. 343–361. Marcel Dekker, New York.

Protocol 10.1

Establishment and monitoring of a microcarrier culture

Materials

Spinner flask (Bellco) 250 ml with a working culture volume of 100 ml

Microcarriers: Cytodex 1, 2 or 3 (Amersham BioSciences) or Cultispher G (Hyclone) 10 g

Dulbecco's phosphate buffered saline (D-PBS)

D-PBS/EDTA: D-PBS + 0.02% EDTA

Trypsin reagent: 0.25% w/v trypsin + 0.02% w/v EDTA

Trypan blue reagent: 0.5% w/v trypan blue in D-PBS

Crystal violet reagent: 0.2 M citric acid, 0.2% w/v crystal violet and 25 w/v Triton X-100

Method to establish a culture

1. Suspend dry microcarriers (10 g) in 500 ml D-PBS.

2. Wash with D-PBS and autoclave.

3. Allow the microcarriers to settle, remove excess D-PBS by decanting and add culture medium to the microcarriers.

4. Inoculate 100 ml culture medium containing 5 mg/ml Cytodex microcarriers with 2×10^5 cells/ml in a spinner flask.

5. Place the spinner flask on a stirrer platform positioned inside a CO_2 incubator and maintain a stirring rate of 50 rpm.

6. Take a sample every day by withdrawing 1 ml of culture and insert into an Eppendorf tube (1.8 ml) for cell counting.

7. Allow the microcarriers to settle and withdraw the supernatant for analysis of medium components.

Counting method 1: trypan blue counting

8. Wash the microcarrier/cell samples with PBS/EDTA and then treat with 1 ml trypsin reagent.

9. Incubate for 10 min at 37°C.

10. Remove the supernatant by Pasteur pipette and add an equal volume of trypan blue (0.5%) to each sample prior to counting cells by hemocytometer.

Counting method 2: crystal violet counting

11. Add an equal volume of crystal violet reagent to the microcarrier/cell pellet.

12. Incubate for 90 min at 37°C.

13. Count the stained nuclei that are released from the microcarriers by hemo-cytometer counting.

Notes

The microcarriers are supplied as a dry powder and are reconstituted in aqueous buffer. Cytodex 1 consists of 4.5×10^6 beads/g dry weight. Cultispher G consists of 0.9×10^6 beads/g dry weight. The dry microcarriers may swell in liquid. The spinner flasks should be siliconized before use to prevent microcarriers sticking on to the glass surface. A siliconizing fluid (dimethyldichlorosilane dissolved in an organic solvent) is used to wet the inner surface of a spinner flask prior to washing and autoclaving. One coating of the siliconizing agent is sufficient for several cycles of use of a spinner flask. Commercially available siliconizing fluids include Sigmacote (Sigma Chemical Co.) and Repelcote (Hopkins and Williams).

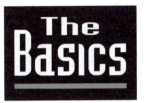

Chapter 11

Production from cell culture

1. Why use animal cell culture for production?

Many healthcare products can be derived from fractionation of blood or extraction from human tissue. However, it is difficult to ensure that such products are free from contamination, particularly by viruses. This risk can be reduced considerably by using well-characterized animal cell lines that are shown to be free of contaminating viruses. As an example, factor VIII used for the treatment of hemophilia was purified from pooled human plasma in the early 1980s. This process was discontinued when samples were found to be contaminated with human immunodeficiency virus (HIV). The safety of the present recombinant product is now ensured by careful screening of the mammalian cell line used in the large-scale bioprocess.

Genetically engineered mammalian cells can overexpress and secrete glycoprotein products into the culture medium. Protein extraction from the culture medium is relatively efficient particularly if a low-protein culture medium is used. In comparison, secretion of protein from genetically engineered bacteria can be more problematic. The synthesized protein usually accumulates as insoluble aggregates within bacterial cells and so requires extraction from the cell lysate. This is more difficult because of the high content of other proteins (including some endotoxins) that must be completely removed from the final product. Thus, the recovery process from the cell lysate is more complex and the final yield of purified product may be lower.

2. How to produce biologicals from cell culture

The first obvious questions to ask before setting up a cell culture process for production are:

- What product do I want?
- How pure do I want it?
- How much do I want?

The type of process, strategy and design will depend upon the answers to these three critical questions.

2.1 What product?

The type of product required is the key to deciding which type of cell to use for production. For simple proteins such as insulin or growth hormone that have low molecular weights and no attached carbohydrate groups, a genetically engineered *Escherichia coli* culture producing the recombinant protein may be preferred. Bacteria grow faster and under more robust conditions than animal cells. However, there are limitations of using bacteria for the expression and production of more complex mammalian proteins. The most serious consideration is that there are a number of post-translational processes that are necessary to modify proteins before they become biologically active:

- proteolytic cleavage;
- subunit association;
- chemical derivatization;
- glycosylation;
- phosphorylation;
- fatty acylation.

In particular, glycosylation has received a lot of attention (Chapter 7). Glycosylation is the intracellular process that involves the addition of a carbohydrate group on to the synthesized protein. The process occurs in the Golgi apparatus prior to secretion through the cell membrane. The carbohydrate component of glycoproteins is often essential for biological activity. Proteins that are under-glycosylated are often cleared from the bloodstream too quickly.

Prokaryotes (such as *E. coli*) are not capable of glycosylation. Yeast cells may be genetically engineered to produce a protein from a transfected mammalian gene. Yeast cells can glycosylate proteins but the carbohydrate added may be different from that in the authentic mammalian glycoprotein and this could influence the therapeutic activity of the molecule.

The carbohydrate content of naturally occurring glycoproteins can vary from 3% (e.g. immunoglobulin) to 40% (e.g. erythropoietin) of the total weight and can be important for many biological properties. Glycoprotein extracted from a culture may be in various glycoforms. These are molecules having an identical protein structure but with differing carbohydrate additives. This type of variation may be unacceptable for some applications, such as for therapeutic use, where a single glycoform may be required. The extent of glycosylation of proteins produced in culture depends on the conditions. The optimal conditions for full glycosylation are often unknown but it has been shown that reduced glycosylation may occur at the end of the growth phase and during the stationary phase of culture.

In most cases, a genetically modified cell line will be required to obtain a specific glycoprotein at a reasonable yield, using the principles described in Chapter 6. The most commonly used host cell lines for such production are Chinese hamster ovary (CHO) and baby hamster kidney (BHK) because their genetics and growth characteristics have been well characterized.

However, in some cases a mammalian cell line may be found that will produce the required glycoprotein product without any genetic manipulation. An example of this is interferon (alpha or beta) production from human fibroblasts. An induction process has been developed which allows high productivity from these cells (see Chapter 12).

The production of animal viruses from cell culture requires some consideration of an acceptable host cell. In this process it is important to know which cell line is susceptible to the particular strain of virus required. Also, the mode of culture may be important. For example, the extent of viral infection is often greater in anchorage-dependent cells attached to a substratum.

2.2 How pure?

If a product is required for human injection – as a therapeutic agent or as a prophylactic viral vaccine – then high standards of purification are needed with an absolute requirement to ensure the absence of known risk factors. If a product is required as a diagnostic agent or for laboratory use, then the conditions of purification may be less stringent. Electrophoresis is a powerful method for discriminating between proteins. Thus the visualization of a single stained protein band by gel electrophoresis is a good indicator of the purity of a protein.

The purity requirements for the final product may influence not only the purification process (downstream processing) chosen but also the conditions of culture. For example, purification is easier if the cell product is secreted into a low-protein or protein-free culture media. Also, it may be necessary to avoid antifoam or shear protective agents as these can foul membrane-based purification processes.

The timing of product harvest may be important because of the risk of product exposure to proteases or glycosidases, that may arise from cell lysis. These enzymes will cause breakdown of the protein backbone or carbohydrate group of a glycoprotein product.

2.3 How much?

Deciding the quantity of cell product required over a set period of time is vital to planning a production process. This is equally important for a laboratory preparation as well as a large-scale commercial enterprise (Thilly, 1986). The importance of this question to developing a process strategy can be best illustrated by an example of the production of a hypothetical glycoprotein (Biolikin).

The biotechnology company, Candogene, planned to make 10 kg of Biolikin from a cell with a product yield of 1 pg/cell-day. Could this requirement for 10^{16} cell-days of production be met by their stirred tank reactor at 10^6 cells/ml? The strategic planners at Candogene determined that this would require a day's run on a 10 million (10^7)-liter fermenter and abandoned the project as beyond their scope.

However, an alternative company decided to take up this project by a three-stage plan.

1. They improved the specific productivity of the cell line ($\times 100$) by gene amplification (see Chapter 6). This reduced the required culture capacity to 10^5 liters.
2. They decided to use a perfusion culture that increased the final cell concentration to 4×10^7/ml. This reduced the required culture capacity to 2500 liters.
3. They decided that there was no need to make the product in 1 day but could continue the process over 100 days. This reduced the required culture capacity to 25 liters, which was well within the fermenter size available in their small laboratory.

This example illustrates that missed opportunities can arise from poor or no planning and by not asking the right questions from the onset of the work.

2.4   The scale of production

Animal cell products generally have a high value but a low demand in terms of quantity. This can be illustrated by figures available for erythropoietin, which is one of the successful recombinant products used as a clinical agent. According to a figure from 1998, the total US demand for this therapeutic agent was satisfied by 1 kilogram per year and the product was sold for $1600/mg. This demand can be accommodated by a 10 000 liter bioreactor with a production level of 500 units/ml after a 10-day period of cell growth. Typically, the specific activity of EPO is 130 000 units/mg.

This principle applies to most animal cell bioprocesses, where the scale of homogeneous suspension cultures is rarely above 10 000 liters and for nonhomogeneous microcarrier cultures rarely above 1000 liters. The three major technical problems of scale up of unit processes are mass transfer, mixing times and shear forces.

- Mass transfer: Oxygen must be provided to meet the metabolic demand of the cells without high stirring rates or intense gas sparging that may cause cell damage. The damaging effect of gas sparging may be reduced by additives such as Pluronic (see Chapter 9).
- Mixing: If the cultures are fed with nutrients then the mixing rate should be adequate to prevent concentration gradients that could damage cells or cause uneven growth.
- Shear forces: If the stirring rates are not too high then the cells will not be damaged by shear forces. However, the stirring rate must be sufficient to allow efficient mixing and mass transfer.

2.5   The type of bioprocess

Most large-scale bioprocesses presently in operation are designed as fed-batch cultures. The advantage is simplicity and ease of scale-up. High cell densities may be obtained if an appropriate mixture of components is fed to the cells at strategic intervals.

The alternative mode of culture that is used in around 10% of bioprocesses involving animal cells is perfusion. This has the advantage of allowing high cell densities by a continuous supply of nutrients and removal of cell-free products from the bioreactor. This removes the products from long contact with the cells that may release degradative enzymes such as proteinases and sialidases. There is a high productivity from such a process and it can be maintained for long periods of time. The disadvantage of the perfusion bioprocess is the high initial starting cost. Because of this, the perfusion mode is best suited for the production of proteins that are required in relatively large quantities (>100 kg/year).

2.6   Alternative methods for multiple products required in small quantity

Monoclonal antibodies are a special category of products because they are required in relatively small amounts but in multiple types with differing antigen specificities. The standard method of production has been injection of hybridomas into the peritoneal cavity of mice. The growth of the hybridoma releases monoclonal antibody into the ascites fluid which can be extracted from the mouse.

The production of monoclonal antibodies by mice has come under increasing criticism because of the ethical issues posed by the use of laboratory animals and particularly given the availability of alternative methods. In most European countries regulatory approval has been withdrawn except when it can be shown that the use of animals is the only means of production. Additionally the ascites method presents problems for product purification. The overall protein content of ascites fluid is high, posing difficulties in obtaining pure monoclonal antibodies. Furthermore, the ascites fluid contains antibodies secreted by the host mouse, which are impossible to separate from the desired monoclonal antibody. Thus the final product following purification may have residual activity that will interfere with the activity of the monoclonal antibody.

In vitro production of monoclonal antibodies can occur by small hollow-fiber bioreactors which can be run continuously for several months. The antibody productivity from such a bioreactor run for 2 months has been shown to be equivalent to the use of around 20 mice. Depending upon the specific productivity of the hybridoma, this would typically produce 100–1000 mg of antibody. A cost analysis shows that these processes are broadly equivalent with a production cost of $1–2 per mg antibody (Jackson *et al.*, 1996).

The hollow-fiber bioreactor is a convenient system for continuous production of small quantities of antibody, although some problems can arise because of the high cell densities that occur. Limited gas diffusion may produce an oxygen deficiency which has been shown to reduce full glycosylation of the secreted immunoglobulin. An alternative is to use a simple small batch culture such as the gas-permeable bags that have been designed from 0.5–2 liters (Lipski *et al.*, 1998).

3. How to purify the final product

The process of purification – often called 'downstream processing' – is dependent on the product and the degree of purification required (Lyddiatt, 1991). However, some general principles can be provided here.

Primary separation involves the removal of cells and debris from the medium. In the case of immobilized cell cultures, this can occur by sedimentation of the cell-loaded particles. For suspension cultures, cells are normally removed by low-speed centrifugation or by filtration. It is important in this primary separation to minimize cell lysis and ensure the removal of all cell debris as this can give rise to degradative enzymes which are capable of causing product breakdown. Chilling the medium (4°C) can also minimize the activity of these enzymes.

Product concentrations arising from a cell culture are generally low – 10–100 mg/l. So, the next stage of purification often involves increasing the concentration by a de-watering process. This can be accomplished by precipitation with a suitable agent such as ethanol, polyethylene glycol or ammonium sulfate. These precipitating agents can be specific for certain protein types and it is important to ensure that the conditions and concentration are appropriate for precipitating the protein required. An alternative method of concentration is by ultrafiltration using a hollow-fiber cartridge, which can concentrate by 10–100-fold. The hollow-fiber cartridge should

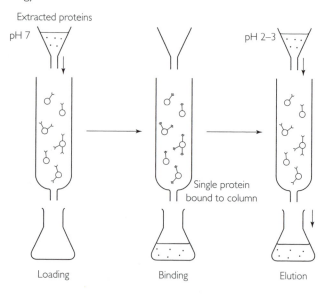

Extracted proteins

pH 7

pH 2–3

Single protein
bound to column

Loading   Binding   Elution

Figure 11.1

Immunoaffinity purification.

have a high-molecular-weight cut-off, so that the product, but not the cells, passes through the fiber. For example, with a 10-kDa cut-off, the concentrated 'retentate' will include all substances above that molecular weight while all lower-molecular-weight substances will be drained off as 'permeate'.

To maximize the yield of the final product extracted from culture media, it is important to have as few purification steps as possible. This can be achieved particularly if highly selective fractionation procedures are available. Bioselective adsorption methods are particularly valuable because of the selectivity for a single compound or group of compounds. For example, Protein A and Protein G have specificity for binding immunoglobulins. Also, monoclonal antibodies are useful because of their affinity for particular compounds.

The adsorption reagents can be prepared by immobilization of an antibody to a solid matrix such as Sepharose. This is suitable for column chromatography because of the open-pore structure which allows a reasonably high liquid flow rate. Reactive forms such as cyanogen bromide-activated Sepharose are available commercially and can be bound covalently to a protein ligand (such as an antibody). *Figure 11.1* shows the principle of immunoaffinity column purification. A protein extract is loaded on to the column at neutral pH, allowing a single protein (the antigen) to bind to the antibody sites. After washing the column with further neutral pH buffer, the antigen is eluted in a pure state with a low pH buffer.

4. The efficiency and productivity of a culture system

The production of biologicals from animal cells is akin to chemical synthesis in which the cells can be considered as catalysts promoting the conversion of relatively simple nutrient molecules into specific complex macromolecules. All genetic or biochemical manipulations of the cells are designed to

convert them into efficient chemical catalysts – a process which may change
the cells significantly from their original state.

Cell products are normally secreted into the culture media by viable
cells. The final yield of the product will depend on:

- the specific productivity of each viable cell – expressed as µg of product
  formed per 10^6 cell-day;
- the viable cell density of the culture ($\times 10^6$ cells/ml).

Productivity can be maximized by ensuring the following.

- The cells selected following transfection have the highest level of product
  synthesis. This may require gene amplification as explained in Chapter 6.
  In some cases selective pressure while the cells are grown may ensure that
  genes are continuously amplified and fully active. In the DHFR amplification system, this may require the inclusion of methotrexate in the
  culture medium and the exclusion of hypoxanthine and thymidine (see
  Chapter 6).
- Cell selection involving repeated cloning is also important for high
  productivity following hybridization of antibody-producing cells (see
  Chapter 8). These procedures will ensure that a cell line will be
  obtained for high protein yields in culture and may make productivity
  differences of as much as 10–100-fold.
- Favorable culture conditions are required to ensure that cells reach a
  high density. The productivity is often independent of cell growth and
  as such the products may be considered to be secondary metabolites.
  This means that productivity will be directly related to the number of
  viable cells in culture and it is an advantage to maintain the cells in a
  viable condition for as long as possible through the growth and stationary phases. This may not be possible for some cells. If cell death
  occurs by apoptosis (see Chapter 4) then the culture phase will shift
  quickly from a growth to a decline phase – a phenomenon typical of
  antibody-secreting hybridomas.

Figure 11.2 shows a typical increase in product concentration during culture.
The monoclonal antibody (Mab) concentration increases to 140 µg/ml over
the 7-day culture period. Notice that in this example production continues
even after the maximum cell density is reached at day 4.

The cell-specific productivity can be measured from these data by first
determining a set of integral values from the growth curve (often called 'the
viability index'):

$$\int_0^t N_v \, dt$$

This is done by measuring the area under the growth plot from time zero to
each cell concentration point. Geometric measurements can be used (tra-
pezoid method) or simple computer programs are available (e.g. Sigmaplot).
The change in product concentration is then plotted against the viability
index and the specific rate of productivity determined from the slope.

$$Q_s = \Delta P \cdot \frac{1}{\int_0^t N_v \, dt}$$

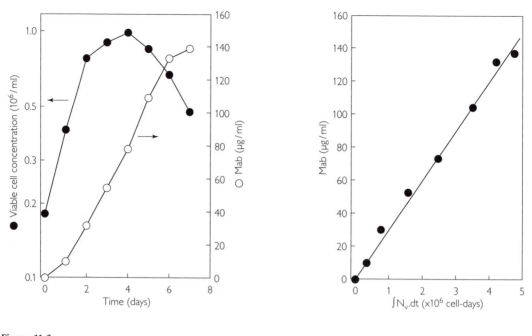

Figure 11.2

Measurement of specific productivity.

This calculation is similar to that used in Chapter 10 for substrate uptake and by-product formation.

The gradient of the resulting straight line is the specific productivity (pg/cell-day or μg/10^6 cell-day). For the generation of some products such as monoclonal antibodies the specific production rate has been found to be constant throughout the culture of hybridomas (Renard *et al.*, 1988). If production is growth related then this will be apparent from the plot by a steep slope during the growth phase. In *Figure 11.2*, the production is independent of the phase of the culture and a productivity of 30 μg/10^6 cell-day can be calculated. Growth-dependent productivity would be indicated by an increased gradient of this plot in the growth phase and then a decreased gradient as cell concentration declines.

The productivity of a cell culture process may be expressed in several ways to give an indication of efficiency. Final cell densities can vary between typical values of 10^6 cells/ml for batch cultures, to 10^7 cells/ml for perfusion, to 10^8 cells/ml for hollow-fiber systems. However, you need to assess such comparisons with care. A higher final cell density in a perfusion or hollow-fiber system may be obtained following the expenditure of a considerable volume of medium. High cell densities may occur only in part of the bio-reactor system such as the extracapillary space of hollow fibers or the interior of cell-entrapping beads. The cell yield per total volume of expended medium may be a more valuable comparison to make between such systems.

However, even this can be misleading as an indicator of the overall process efficiency and it is important to consider all the factors involved in the production process. For example, a product released into a low-protein medium may eventually be extracted more efficiently than one released into a high-serum medium. This can have an important bearing on the economics of the production process. Thus, the ultimate indicator of the efficiency of an overall process is the total operation cost per unit weight of the purified product.

5.   Cost of the cell culture process

A cost analysis of a commercial operation involving animal cells will take into account various factors including labor, materials and capital cost. Generally the unit cost of production decreases with scale-up. This is usually an indication of a significant decrease in the labor cost as a percentage of the total unit cost. This is because the demands of managing a 1000-liter fermenter are less than 10 times that of a 100-liter fermenter – a fact that shows the value of a unit process as compared with multiple processes where the number of manipulations increases proportionally to the number of cultures in operation.

Figure 11.3 shows a typical cost analysis of a commercial operation involving antibody production from airlift fermenters in Celltech, UK. Here the advantage of scale-up is shown by a dramatic decrease in the unit cost of the product with a ×100 increase in scale. Thus, 1 mg of Mab produced in a 10 000-liter bioreactor would cost 90% less than the equivalent cost in a 100-liter bioreactor. In *Figure 11.3b* the production cost is broken into three components: labor, consumable materials and equipment depreciation. At the smaller scale the labor cost is the major component of the total

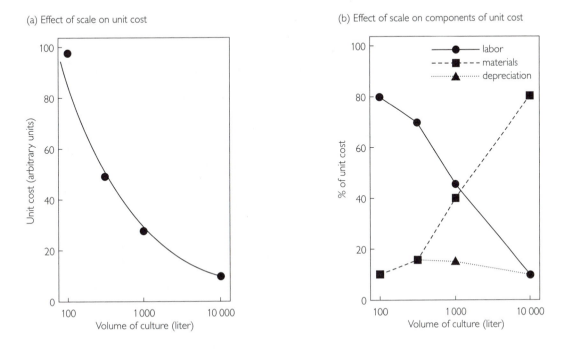

(a) Effect of scale on unit cost

(b) Effect of scale on components of unit cost

Figure 11.3

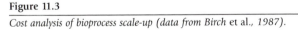

Cost analysis of bioprocess scale-up (data from Birch et al., *1987).*

production cost. However, this decreases dramatically with increase in the scale of operation, from 80 to 10% of the unit cost in the example.

On the other hand, material costs increase substantially as a proportion of the total cost during scale-up. This suggests that any saving in the cost of materials, such as the growth medium, could have a significant effect in lowering the unit cost of a product of a large-scale process.

In order to reduce media costs, several approaches may be considered. Omission of antibiotics, use of a lowered serum content or use of an alternative to fetal calf serum would permit significant cost reductions. Fetal calf serum can account for as much as 90% of the total medium cost. Serum-free media formulations may be suitable for the growth of specific cell lines although these formulations may contain certain hormones and growth factors, the combined cost of which may exceed that of the serum supplement. However, a serum-free formulation may still be justified in a large-scale operation if there are benefits in product purification.

The optimization of the cell culture strategy can increase productivity and can offer an alternative to increasing culture volume. The choice of media perfusion rather than batch culture can lead to significant increases in cell yields (see Chapter 10). Continuous cultures generally have a higher productivity than batch cultures. Although perfusion may require the expenditure of larger volumes of medium, it may be possible to use diluted media or carefully controlled dilution rates to improve overall productivity. The formulation of optimal growth media or the development of a regime of selected nutrient addition and inhibitor removal may lead to routinely higher cell yields. Considerations of this sort in planning culture operations may significantly alter the economics of a process and reduce the overall unit cost of the final product.

References

Birch, J.R., Thompson, P.W., Boraston, R., Oliver, S. and Lambert, K. (1987) The large-scale production of monoclonal antibodies in airlift fermenters. In: Webb, C. and Mavituna, F. (eds) *Plant and Animal Cells: Process Possibilities*, pp. 162–171. Ellis Horwood, Chichester.

Jackson, L.R., Trudel, L.J., Fox, J.G. and Lipman, N.S. (1996) Evaluation of hollow fiber bioreactors as an alternative to murine ascites production for small scale monoclonal antibody production. *J. Immunol. Methods* **189**: 217–231.

Lipski, L.A., Witzleb, M.P., Reddington, G.M. and Reddington, J.J. (1998) Evaluation of small to moderate scale in vitro monoclonal antibody production via the use of the iMAb gas-permeable bag system. *Res. Immunol.* **149**: 547–552.

Lyddiatt, A. (1991) Downstream processing: protein recovery. In: Butler, M. (ed.) *Mammalian Cell Biotechnology: A Practical Approach*, pp.187–206. IRL Press at Oxford University Press, Oxford.

Renard, J.M., Spagnoli, R., Mazier, C., Salles, M.F. and Mandine, E. (1988) Evidence that monoclonal antibody production kinetics is related to the integral of the viable cell curve in batch systems. *Biotechnol. Let.* **10**: 91–96.

Thilly, W.G. (1986) The rationale for and elements of mammalian cell technology. In: Thilly, W.G. (ed.) *Mammalian Cell Technology*, pp 1–8. Butterworth, Boston.

Further reading

Vinci, V.A. and Parekh, S.R. (2003) *Handbook of Industrial Cell Culture*. Humana Press, New Jersey.

Chapter 12

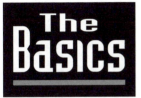

Mammalian cell products: established and potential

1. Introduction

Animal cells synthesize a vast range of compounds that can be extracted and purified from cultures. Many of these compounds have potential value as healthcare products. The initial challenge for the clinical application of these products is to isolate a sufficient quantity at an acceptable level of purity. This involves the culture and scale-up procedures outlined in Chapters 9 and 10.

There have been three major innovations in the development of mammalian cell cultures for the production of biologicals in the last few decades. Each has led to the production of a new category of biologicals.

- Viral vaccines: from the ability to grow viruses in cell culture.
- Monoclonal antibodies: from the ability to generate hybridomas by cell fusion. These were considered in Chapter 8.
- Recombinant proteins: from the ability to transfect cells with isolated genes and amplify to allow high level of expression of the corresponding proteins.

The use of these products in human clinical applications will be discussed in this chapter. Expansion of specific cell lines has been used in such areas as toxicity testing and various clinical procedures. The applications of these cell products will also be discussed in this chapter.

2. Viral vaccines

Enders discovered in 1949 that the poliomyelitis virus could be grown from primary monkey cells in culture. The virus has an icosahedron structure with an inner core of nucleic acid and an outer coat or capsid which is made of repeated protein capsomere structures (*Figure 12.1*). The polio vaccine, produced in 1954, was the first human vaccine to be produced using large-scale cell culture techniques. This eventually led to the development of animal cell technology for the production of a range of human and veterinary viral vaccines against a variety of diseases (*Table 12.1*). This offers a more consistent and efficient method of production compared to alternatives such as the propagation of virus in chick embryos, a method that has been used even up to recent times.

Childhood vaccination is now routine and the importance of these vaccines in the improvement of world health over the last half century has been enormous. Polio vaccines exist as inactivated viruses (Salk) or live attenuated viruses (Sabin). Both have been used extensively throughout the world with the result that incidence of poliomyelitis is now extremely low in the West.

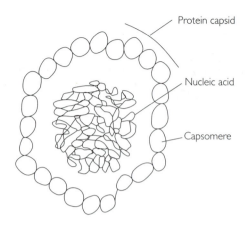

Figure 12.1

An icosahedron virus particle.

Table 12.1. Examples of virus vaccines produced in large quantities

Human	Veterinary
Polio	Foot-and-mouth disease
Measles	Marek's disease
Mumps	Newcastle disease
Rubella	Rinderpest
Yellow fever	Rabies
Rabies	Canine distemper
Influenza	Swine fever
	Blue tongue
	Fowl pox

Smallpox was completely eradicated as a world disease in the 1960s and now has only arisen as a potential weapon of bioterrorism from the culture stocks that were retained in specific designated laboratories. Both of these diseases were at one time endemic and widespread, particularly among the young.

The basis of vaccination is to inject a viral antigen in a nonpathogenic form. This induces the formation of a corresponding antibody which can provide some protection against the live virus and the associated disease. The two major vaccine types are listed below.

■   An inactivated pathogenic virus. This is a disease-causing virus which has been chemically inactivated.

■   An attenuated live virus. This is capable of propagation but has been changed genetically so that it can not produce a disease. However, the virus still has the surface proteins capable of eliciting an immune response which protects against the pathogenic virus. Live viral vaccines are often preferred because they can be administered in small but effective doses.

2.1   Production of viruses

Animal viruses can be propagated by inoculation into a culture of cells at relatively high density. The cell type should be susceptible to the particular virus required. Anchorage-dependent cell growth is particularly well suited for viral growth and for large-scale production, with microcarrier cultures often being used.

The typical events associated with viral infection of a cell culture are shown in *Figure 12.2*. The lytic cycle consists of four distinct phases of adsorption, penetration, replication and release. During this cycle, cellular metabolism is directed to the formation of new virus particles and eventual cell lysis. However, some viruses do not cause cell lysis but arise by budding from the cell membrane.

The quantity of virus is usually expressed in plaque-forming units (pfu) which relates to the formation of a plaque on a monolayer of cells. The plaque is recognized under a microscope by a clear spot in the monolayer caused by cell lysis as a result of infection by a single virus. A plaque assay involves addition of a virus suspension at various dilutions to cell mono-layers in a series of Petri dishes. The pfu values are determined from counts on the Petri dishes in which distinct and separate plaques can be distinguished.

For production the virus is added to a cell culture at a multiplicity of infection (moi) of $0.1-10$ pfu/cell with the expectation that this will increase to 10^3-10^4 pfu/cell following a period of propagation. This represents an increase of up to $\times 10^5$ of the total virus in the culture. It is important to iden-tify the time of maximum titer of extracellular virus. This normally occurs about 12–24 hours after viral inoculation and is the time at which the viruses should be harvested and purified from the culture (see *Figure 12.3*).

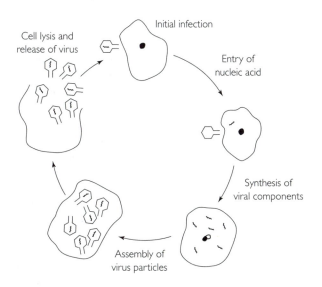

Figure 12.2

Lytic cycle of viral infection.

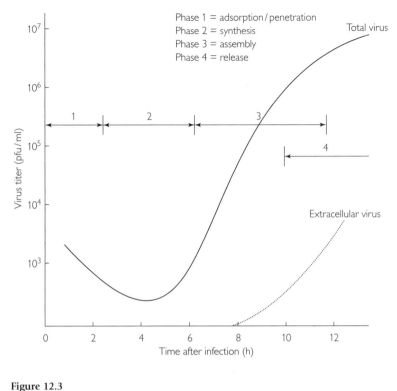

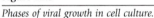

Figure 12.3

Phases of viral growth in cell culture.

The outline given here is intended only as a brief guide to the events associated with viral infection and production. For specific details related to a particular virus and the possibilities for production, see, for example Mahy (1985).

2.2 Cell lines for vaccine production

Safety is of major concern when choosing a cell line for vaccine production. During the development of vaccine production processes, it was decided that the perceived risk of using tumorigenic cell lines such as the well-characterized HeLa cells as a substrate for viral propagation was unacceptable. In 1954 the regulatory bodies in the USA decreed that human vaccines should be produced from primary cells derived from healthy monkeys. The poliomyelitis vaccine was subsequently produced by viral propagation on primary monkey kidney cells. However, it was discovered later that these cells were contaminated with a newly discovered tumorigenic virus designated SV40. This caused concern even though there was no evidence for the transmission of the SV40 virus to recipients of the vaccine.

Extensive study and characterization of normal human diploid fibroblasts in the early 1960s led to their acceptance for vaccine production. Two human lung fibroblast lines named WI-38 and MRC-5 have now been used extensively for polio vaccine production. Even though these cells have a finite lifespan, their use in the large-scale propagation of viruses is much easier than the alternative of obtaining primary cells for each batch of vaccines. Consequently, large stocks of these human cell lines at low passage number have been maintained for use in vaccine production. The capacity for vaccine production from an individual strain is enormous despite the finite limit on propagation.

Vero (African green monkey cells) was the first continuous cell line to be accepted as a substrate for human vaccine production and polio vaccine has been produced from these cells in France since 1983. This is a continuous cell line with excellent growth characteristics. Despite its heteroploid genetic character it has not been shown to be tumorigenic.

A live virulent virus requires complete inactivation before it can be used as a vaccine. Treatment with formaldehyde can be effective providing the treatment is for a sufficient time to ensure inactivation of all virus particles.

An alternative vaccine is the live attenuated virus. This has the antigenic determinants of the normal virus but has been modified genetically so that it is no longer pathogenic. The attenuation can be induced by mutagenic agents but in most cases it occurs spontaneously by continuous passage of the virus in cell culture. Vaccines can also be produced as peptides which mimic the antigenic effect of the viral coat protein.

3. Monoclonal antibodies

The background and practical methods associated with the development of monoclonal antibodies (Mabs) are described in Chapter 8. All useful applications of monoclonal antibodies depend upon their high specificity of binding to an antigen. Many Mabs produced commercially are used for diagnostic tests for the identification of small quantities of specific antigens. Changes in the level of hormones or enzymes in blood or urine can be used to check for pregnancy or any change of physiological state. Immunodiagnostic tests of this type can be performed within 15–20 min, which has considerable benefit for the early diagnosis and in the treatment of disease.

3.1 Therapeutic antibodies

Mabs also have applications as therapeutic agents, particularly in targeted drug therapy (James, 1990). In 1986 the monoclonal antibody named OKT3 developed by Ortho Pharmaceuticals was the first murine Mab to be licensed for therapeutic use. OKT3 recognizes a surface antigen (CD3) on T-lymphocytes and is one of the most effective agents in preventing immunological rejection of transplanted kidneys. Of course, therapeutic Mabs take a longer time to develop because of the need for the strict clinical trials that are required before any injectable compound can be licensed for human treatment. Clinical trials that demonstrate safety are often the most costly part of developing a new medicinal product.

Various monoclonal antibodies have been targeted to membrane-bound protein antigens specifically expressed in tumor cells. These antibodies can be designed in configurations likely to cause the destruction of the target tumor cells. The conjugation of radioactive or toxic compounds to the antibody can result in a localized high concentration resulting in cytotoxicity to the target cells. Alternatively, an enzyme may be conjugated that will catalyze the release of a toxic product from an ingested 'pro-drug'. Another strategy is to promote an effector function through the use of a bispecific antibody that could potentially activate T-cells leading to the specific destruction of the target cells.

The rationale behind these methods is to cause localized cell destruction but limit systemic toxicity. However, the results of the initial clinical trials for therapeutic murine antibodies using these strategies were disappointing. This was as a result of unexpected toxicity associated with treatment of immuno-conjugates and the undesirable human anti-murine antibody (HAMA) immune response. However, the administration of antibodies relying on a response within a short period of time (up to 10 days) was more successful. This included antibodies for radioimaging, radioimmunotherapy or for acute allograft rejection (the OKT3 antibody).

The development of human chimeric antibodies in the 1990s increased rapidly the rate of licensing of monoclonal antibodies as therapeutic agents. These humanized antibodies do not elicit the HAMA effect and also the half-life is much longer than mouse antibodies. Most mouse IgGs have a half-life of less than 20 h whereas an antibody with a human-type constant region can have a half-life of up to 21 days. *Table 12.2* shows eight monoclonal antibodies that have been approved recently by the USA regulatory agency, the FDA, for human therapeutic use. As well as these, there are many more antibodies in clinical trials with the expectation that the numbers in therapeutic use will increase in the future (von Mehren *et al.*, 2003).

The success of these chimeric antibodies can be illustrated by Rituxan which is used in the treatment of non-Hodgkin's lymphoma. This has a murine variable region which binds specifically to CD20 on B-cells and a human Fc domain to trigger effector mechanisms. CD20 is a protein expressed by over 90% of the lymphoma cells. These tumor cells can become coated by the anti-CD20. This results in activation of the complement pathway and Fc receptor-bearing cells which can destroy the tumor cell.

Table 12.2. Monoclonal antibodies approved by the FDA for clinical use

Antibody	Type	Therapeutic treatment	Company	Date approved
Orthoclone (OKT3)	Murine Ig2a	Allograft rejection	Ortho Biotech	1986
ReoPro	Chimeric (Fab)	Coronary angioplasty	Centocor/Lilly	1994
Zenapax	Humanized IgG1	Allograft rejection	Protein Design/ Hoffman-La Roche	1997
Rituxan	Chimeric IgG1	Non-Hodgkin's lymphoma	Genentech	1997
Synagis	Humanized IgG1	Respiratory syncytial virus	Medimmune	1998
Herceptin	Humanized IgG1	Breast cancer	Genentech	1998
Simulect	Chimeric IgG1	Allograft rejection	Novartis Pharm	1998
Inflixmab	Chimeric IgG1	Rheumatoid arthritis/ Crohn's disease	Centocor	1998–1999

4. Therapeutic recombinant glycoproteins from mammalian cells

Proteins extracted from biological sources have been important for substitution therapy since the 1920s when Best and Banting used insulin to treat diabetes. Examples of some of these clinical agents are shown in *Figure 12.4*. However, the problems associated with such extraction processes include the large quantity of tissue, blood or urine required for extraction of the small amount of each product (*Figure 12.5*). In some cases the problem could be solved by extraction from nonhuman sources, although this always poses the risk of an adverse immune response in human recipients. In the case of insulin this was solved by the chemical transformation of pig insulin which differs from the human version only by one amino acid (*Figure 12.6*). However, the overriding reason for abandoning most of these extraction

Protein	Source
• Insulin	Pancreas; bovine or porcine
• Growth hormone	Human pituitary glands
• Interferon	Viral activation of cells
• Urokinase	Human urine
• Factor VIII	Pooled human blood

Figure 12.4

Products extracted from tissue/primary cells.

- Small quantities available
- Nonhuman proteins cause immunogenicity
- Contamination with viruses or prions
    - Creutzfeld-Jakob disease
    - HIV from blood

Figure 12.5

Problems of extraction from animal/human sources.

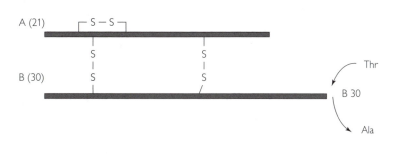

Figure 12.6

Pig to human insulin.

processes is the risk of contamination from infectious agents such as HIV and prions.

In this section, the background of the development of processes for the commercial production of glycoproteins secreted from genetically engineered mammalian cell lines will be described (Lubiniecki and Lupker, 1994). In most cases these are natural products that can be produced in large quantities following the isolation of a specific gene which is then expressed in a host cell line.

4.1 Interferons

In 1957 Isaacs and Lindenmann discovered a compound that 'interfered' with viral propagation in cells in culture and introduced the term interferon. They showed that culture medium taken from cells that had supported viral growth could protect noninfected cells from a subsequent viral infection (Isaacs and Lindenmann, 1957). This led to the identification of a group of proteins that were shown to interfere with the propagation of viruses and subsequently named 'interferons'.

An interferon refers to an inducible secretory protein produced by eukaryotic cells in response to viral and other stimuli. The interferons are now recognized as a family of cytokines having antiviral, antiproliferative and immunoregulatory effects.

The basis of the antiviral activity protecting noninfected cells is illustrated in *Figure 12.7*. Viral infection induces the synthesis of interferon by derepression of the gene. The secreted interferon can then induce an 'antiviral state' in neighboring cells. The molecular mechanism of interferon protection is not fully understood but is thought to involve the synthesis of a number of enzymes including those capable of degrading viral RNA and inhibiting protein synthesis.

The therapeutic value of the interferons is based on their antiviral activity and also on the ability to retard the growth of tumor cells. There are a number of viral infections and cancers that can be effectively treated by use of one of the interferon types.

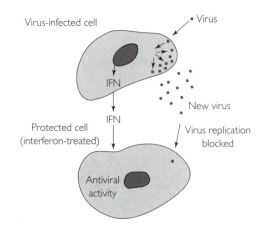

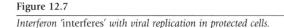

Figure 12.7

Interferon 'interferes' with viral replication in protected cells.

The interferons are a group of relatively small proteins that contain 140–170 amino acids and are divided into three main types – IFN-α, IFN-β and IFN-γ. A further complexity arises in that there are at least 25 independent subtypes of IFN-α which are all products of independent genes. Each interferon type is derived and secreted predominantly by one cell type – B-lymphocytes (IFN-α), fibroblasts (IFN-β) and T-lymphocytes (IFN-γ) – and this accounts for differences in production processes.

IFN-α

A procedure for the isolation of IFN-α from leukocytes obtained from pooled human blood was pioneered in the 1960s but the yield from this process was too low to satisfy the growing demand for interferon. Subsequently a large-scale cell culture production process was developed by Wellcome (UK) to operate in 10 000-liter batch fermenters. This process is based on a human B-lymphoblastoid cell line (Namalwa) that is a particularly good producer of IFN-α following induction with Sendai virus (Lazar, 1983).

The cells grow well in suspension and have been adapted to low-cost serum-free medium. This is one of the few examples of the use of a human transformed cell line for the production of a therapeutic compound. In fact IFN-α was the first product from a tumor cell line to be licensed for human therapy. Improved purification techniques and sensitive assays for DNA can ensure negligible contamination. On this basis IFN-α derived from Namalwa cells has gained approval for routine use in selected life-threatening conditions (e.g. leukemia).

IFN-β

IFN-β and IFN-α2 are the only human interferons that are naturally glycosylated. Naturally occurring human interferon-β is a glycoprotein with an apparent molecular weight of 25 kDa. The peptide structure has 166 amino acid residues and has a molecular weight of 17.5 kDa (corresponding to the nonglycosylated form). The predominant glycan structure of HuIFN-β consists of a biantennary complex-type structure attached to Asn-80.

Human interferon-β is secreted by fibroblasts in response to viral infection or to double-stranded RNA. The physiological mode of action of HuIFN-β is not well understood. Interaction with a cell surface receptor causes the activation of a signal cascade that can affect the transcription of a number of specific genes. *In vitro* studies have shown the ability of HuIFN-β to induce or suppress over 20 gene products. Its beneficial effect as a therapy for multiple sclerosis is ascribed to one of the following: (a) regulation of T-cell function; (b) modulation of production of cytokines causing anti-inflammatory effects; (c) regulation of T-cell migration and infiltration.

Human interferon-β has antiviral and antiproliferative properties and has been used in chemotherapy in the treatment of certain types of solid tumors. However, results of this type of treatment have been disappointing. Pharmacokinetic evidence indicates that the problem might be the short half-life of HuIFN-β in the bloodstream, suggesting that poor performance in cancer trials may be caused by lack of sustained delivery to the tumor site. A solution to this limitation of delivery may be the use of gene therapy to the tumor site (Qin *et al.*, 1998).

HuIFN-β was originally produced from large-scale cultures of human foreskin fibroblasts (such as FS-4) by a process termed 'superinduction' which involves induction with a synthetic polynucleotide (such as polyI:polyC) followed by a regime of antibiotic addition to maximize the stimulation of interferon synthesis (Clark and Hirtenstein, 1981). The rationale behind the superinduction process is to decrease the cellular concentration of an inducible protein repressor which normally causes the breakdown of interferon mRNA. The absence of the repressor can increase (×4) the half-life of IFN mRNA. The overall effect of this is to delay the synthesis of IFN-β but to increase the total productivity 100-fold. The fibroblast cells are generally grown in microcarrier cultures to support growth to high cell densities. This is a procedure adopted by several companies with production occurring in large-scale batch cultures (up to 4000 liters).

In 1993 the use of recombinant HuIFN-β was approved in the treatment of multiple sclerosis (MS). This is a chronic inflammatory disease of the central nervous system that is autoimmune in origin. The result is a deterioration of nerve cells due to a T-lymphocyte-associated breakdown of the myelin sheath of the nerves. HuIFN-β has been shown in clinical trials to reduce the progression of MS in patients. This created renewed interest in the production of interferon. The isolation of the HuIFN-β gene allowed the construction of genetically engineered E. coli and CHO cells for enhanced productivity of the protein. The specific productivity from these transfected cell lines is much greater than from the previously used superinduction process.

There are currently three recombinant HuIFN-β preparations available for MS treatment – Betaseron (HuIFN-β1b), Avonex (HuIFN-β1a) and Rebif (HuIFN-β1a). Betaseron, which was approved in 1993 to treat relapsing, remitting MS, is a nonglycosylated form of recombinant HuIFN-β with a deletion of Met-1 and a Cys-17 to Ser mutation and produced in E. coli. The other two products (Avonex and Rebif) are both glycosylated forms of HuIFN-β produced from transfected Chinese hamster ovary (CHO) cells in culture.

There are several recognized advantages of using the glycosylated HuIFN-β (type-1a) compared to the nonglycosylated form (type-1b). Firstly, it has higher biological activity. Avonex has been shown to have a ×10 higher specific activity than Betaseron in three separate functional assays based on antiviral, antiproliferative and immunomodulatory properties (Runkel et al., 1998). This allows a lower patient dosage (30 μg weekly for Avonex against 250 μg every other day for Betaseron). Secondly, there is a significantly lower production of neutralizing antibodies against the glycosylated form of the molecule (Brickelmaier et al., 1999). Up to 42% of patients treated with Betaseron become positive for neutralizing activity after 3 months as opposed to only 6% of Avonex-treated patients after 12 months.

Kagawa et al. (1988) analyzed the sugar chains of rHuIFN-β derived from three different mammalian cell lines. rHuIFN-β derived from other transfected cell lines (mouse epithelial, C127 and human adenocarcinoma, PC8) show greater differences in glycan structure compared to normal HuIFN-β and CHO-derived rHuIFN-β. In particular, Galα1-3Galβ1-4GlcNAc structures present from C127 and PC8 cells are absent in normal and CHO-derived HuIFN-β (Kagawa et al., 1988).

CHO cell-derived rHuIFN-β showed the greatest similarity to natural HuIFN-β. The proportion of biantennary complex structure was slightly lower

(68%) than analyzed in natural HuIFN-β with a slightly higher proportion of triantennary forms. This compares with a corresponding value of 95% biantennary analyzed by Contradt *et al.* (1987) in CHO-derived rHuIFN-β. The close similarity in structure between the natural and recombinant forms is important to ensure against adverse immunogenicity following long-term clinical treatment.

IFN-γ

Synthesis of natural IFN-γ by T-lymphocytes can be stimulated by a range of antigens or mitogens. The most widely used inducer is staphylococcal enterotoxin A which can stimulate the extracellular release of IFN-γ by human peripheral blood lymphocytes obtained from donors. However, significantly higher productivity of IFN-γ has been obtained from recombinant mammalian cells transfected with the isolated gene. Transfected CHO cells have been used for the large-scale production of IFN-γ (Scahill *et al.*, 1983). Interferon secreted from a recombinant cell is a single subtype, whereas primary cells secrete a heterogeneous mixture of subtypes.

4.2   Plasminogen activators

Thrombosis is one of the major causes of premature death in the Western world. This occurs by the deposition of fibrin in the circulatory system which results in a blockage of blood flow. Under normal physiological conditions the formation of fibrin is controlled by the clotting cascade which is activated during wound healing. The clotting cascade is in equilibrium with the process of fibrinolysis, which is a cascade of reactions culminating in the proteolytic cleavage of fibrin as shown in *Figure 12.8* and which should prevent the undesirable formation of fibrin clots in the bloodstream.

Several structural domains of the t-PA molecule are shown in *Figure 12.9*. These include the 'kringle' domain characterized by looped structures held together by three disulfide bridges. The EGF domain is so named because of an amino acid sequence similar to one found in epidermal growth factor. The 'finger' domain is important in binding to fibrin whilst the serine protease domain contains the active site for proteolytic cleavage.

The large-scale production process of tissue plasminogen activator (t-PA) was originally developed by Genentech (Lubiniecki *et al.*, 1989) and involves synthesis from transfected CHO-K1 cells. High specific rates of production were obtained from these cells by the incorporation of strong

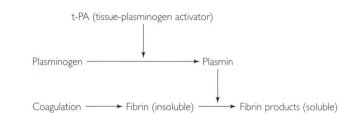

Figure 12.8

Fibrinolysis.

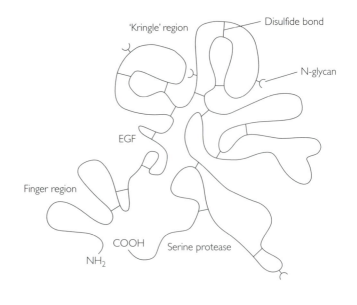

'Kringle' region
Disulfide bond
N-glycan
EGF
Finger region
COOH
Serine protease
NH$_2$

Figure 12.9

Structure of t-PA.

promoters for the transfected gene (see Chapter 6). In 1987, t-PA was one of the first recombinant products derived from mammalian cell culture to be approved for human therapy. For this regulatory approval it was necessary to show that each batch of cultures in the production process produced a consistent yield of t-PA and with the same degree of glycosylation. The final purity of t-PA from this process exceeds 99%.

The effectiveness of this t-PA has been compared with alternative compounds with plasminogen activator properties. These are streptokinase (produced from *Streptomyces*) and urokinase (extracted from urine). Clinical trials have shown that the higher specificity of t-PA for fibrin translates into positive benefits in the treatment of cardiovascular disease.

4.3   Blood-clotting factors

Hemophilia is a sex-linked genetic disease which is characterized by an inactive clotting cascade in the blood. This results in an inability to form fibrin which is necessary for wound healing. The most common forms of clotting disorders of this type are hemophilia A and B which are caused by the absence of factors VIII and IX respectively (Lawn and Vehar, 1986). The role of these factors in the blood-clotting cascade is shown in *Figure 12.10*.

Therapeutic treatment has been performed routinely since the 1940s by regular administration of the appropriate factors to hemophiliacs. The clotting factors have been prepared as concentrates derived from the large-scale fractionation of pooled human blood plasma. Although this approach was successful for a number of years, the use of pooled blood sources is vulnerable to contamination with viruses such as hepatitis B and HIV. Although these viruses can be screened for and inactivated in human blood, the problems have encouraged the search for alternative sources of purified factors VIII and IX.

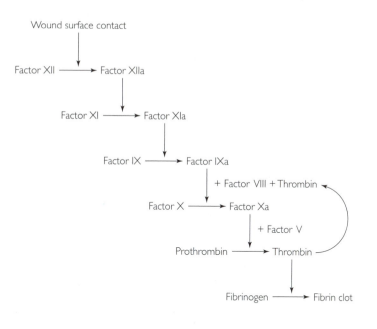

Figure 12.10

The blood-clotting cascade.

Factor VIII

This is a large complex glycoprotein (Mr = 265 kDa). In 1984 the gene for factor VIII was cloned, which was a significant achievement because of the size of the gene (Wood *et al.*, 1984). The factor VIII gene is 186 kilobases long and consists of 26 exons and 25 introns. The cloning involved the ligation of a series of overlapping DNA fragments prepared from genomic and cDNA libraries, aligned to correspond to the full length of the gene, but without introns. Of particular significance in this strategy was the construction of a genomic DNA library from an abnormal human lymphoblastoid cell line with a karyotype containing four copies of the X-chromosome. Because the factor VIII gene is located on the X-chromosome this cell line is enriched with the required gene.

Transfection of a mammalian kidney cell line (BHK) with an expression vector containing the constructed gene allowed synthesis of the biologically active molecule with the correct tertiary folding and glycosylation. The recombinant factor VIII secreted by these cells can be stabilized by the addition of von Willebrand factor. The two factors are normally found as a combined protein complex in blood plasma and are both essential for blood clotting *in vivo*.

The large-scale process for factor VIII production presently operated by Bayer involves the use of a BHK cell line containing approximately 150 copies of the factor VIII gene per cell. The bioprocess involves continuous perfusion over 6 months using a cell retention system similar to those described in Chapter 10. Purification of factor VIII involves anion exchange, immunoaffinity and gel filtration combined with a viral inactivation step. The immunoaffinity chromatography is highly selective for factor VIII but subsequent steps of purification are necessary to ensure the complete removal of any monoclonal antibodies that could leach from the column.

Factor IX

Factor IX is a plasma glycoprotein (Mr = 57 kDa) secreted *in vivo* by hepatocytes. This is also known as Christmas factor, named after the first family diagnosed with the clotting deficiency. The gene for factor IX was originally cloned in 1982. Because the protein requires glycosylation and γ-carboxylation for full activity, a rat hepatoma cell line was used for expression of the gene. This cell line contains the enzymes for the post-translation modifications and was found to be an efficient one for the synthesis of recombinant factor IX (Anson *et al.*, 1985).

4.4   Erythropoietin

The kidney is the source of synthesis of the glycoprotein hormone, erythropoietin (EPO), which is required to ensure continuous red blood cell production in the bone marrow (erythropoiesis) (Eridani, 1990). The absence of EPO in the bloodstream which may be caused by kidney failure will result in the impairment of red blood cell production and consequently, anemia. This condition is treatable by administration of exogenous EPO. Elevated levels of EPO may also be required after extensive blood loss.

EPO is a glycoprotein (Mr = 30–35 kDa) consisting of a 165 amino acid polypeptide chain, two disulfide bonds, three N-linked glycans at Asn-24, -38 and -83 as well as one O-linked glycan at Ser-126 (*Figure 12.11*). The unusually high proportion of carbohydrate (40% by weight) forms a significant component of the overall structure of the molecule as can be seen from the three-dimensional projections of the nonglycosylated and glycosylated molecules shown in *Figure 12.12*. The carbohydrate component is important for full activity *in vivo*. Partially glycosylated EPO is less effective clinically because it is removed rapidly from circulation by specific receptors present in the liver. CHO cells transfected with an expression vector containing the EPO gene have been produced by Amgen (USA) (Goto *et al.*, 1988). The resulting recombinant EPO is effective in the treatment of anemia associated with chronic kidney failure and was licensed for clinical use in 1988. This recombinant hormone has now been extremely successful in the treatment of patients with chronic kidney failure that results in anemia.

The bioactivity of EPO is based upon the binding of a portion of the peptide structure with specific receptors on the surface of the red blood progenitor cells in the bone marrow. Although the glycan component does not affect this interaction directly, it is important to ensure adequate residence time in the bloodstream. Each of the N-glycans can be tetra-sialylated and the O-glycan may be di-sialylated giving a maximum of 14 sialic acid groups per EPO molecule. This results in a low pI (= 4.0). It has been shown that a reduction in the sialylation of EPO causes a proportional decrease in the serum half-life as a result of the removal of the glycoprotein from the circulation by the asialoglycoprotein receptor in the liver.

Egrie and Browne (2001) recently developed a novel form of EPO designated darbepoetin alfa or novel erythropoiesis-stimulating protein (NESP). This is a hyperglycosylated form of recombinant EPO in which two new N-glycan sites were introduced into the molecule by site-directed mutagenesis

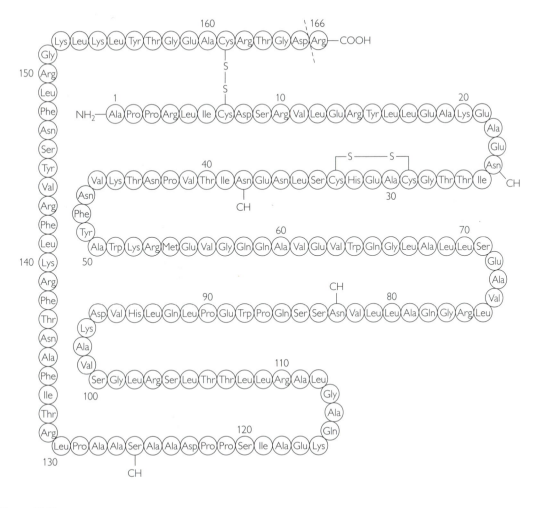

Figure 12.11

Structure of erythropoietin.

at amino acid positions 30 and 88 (*Figure 12.13*). Each of the additional N-glycans increases the molecular weight of the glycoprotein by approximately 3.3 kDa and may contribute up to four additional sialic acids. Thus, the molecular weight of NESP is 37.1 kDa with a maximum of 22 sialic acid groups and a pI of 3.3. The other structures shown in *Figure 12.13* are glycoforms of EPO containing bi-, tri- or tetra-antennary glycans.

Through clinical trials it was shown that the serum half-life of NESP is 26.3 h, which is about 3-fold greater than rEPO. *Figure 12.14* shows the relative increase in serum half-life of three forms of EPO:

■   rEPO (three N-glycans);
■   an analog with four N-glycans;
■   NESP.

Even though the binding capacity of EPO to its receptor decreases with sialylation, the net effect is to enhance the biological activity *in vivo*. This is shown by the gradual increase in the red blood cell count (hematocrit) of

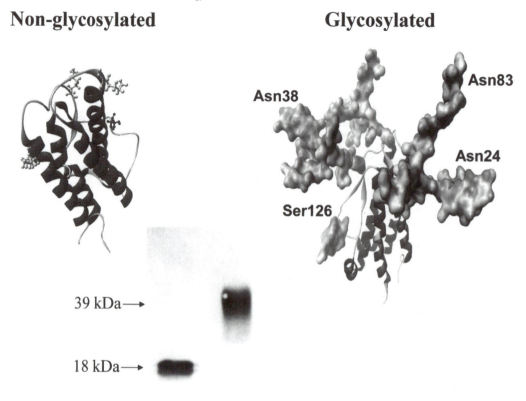

Non-glycosylated   **Glycosylated**

Asn38   Asn83

Asn24

Ser126

39 kDa→

18 kDa→

Figure 12.12

Recombinant human erythropoietin. (Structures kindly provided by Max Crispin and Mark Wormwald.)

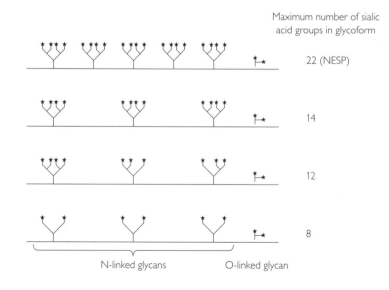

Maximum number of sialic
acid groups in glycoform

22 (NESP)

14

12

8

N-linked glycans   O-linked glycan

Figure 12.13

Variant glycoforms of recombinant EPO and NESP.

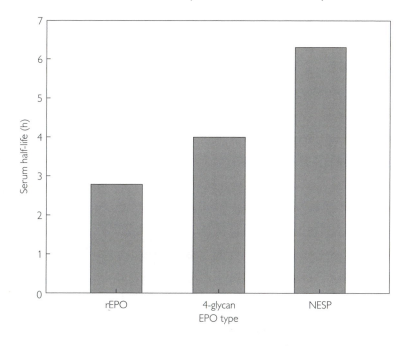

Figure 12.14

Serum half-life of analogs of EPO with variable N-glycan sites.

three groups of mice, each treated for 30 days with one of the EPO isoforms containing a specific number of sialic acids (*Figure 12.15*). The most effective therapeutic isoform of EPO has the highest number of sialic acids. The value of NESP as a therapeutic agent is that the frequency of administration to patients can be decreased significantly for the same clinical effect. However, there is still some uncertainty over the long-term immunogenic response to NESP, which is possible because of the altered amino acid sequence.

5. Risks associated with cell culture products

There are important safety considerations and risk factors that must be considered before a biological product is accepted for clinical use (Lubiniecki, 1987; Petricciani, 1987). There are four main identifiable risk factors associated with animal cell-derived products. The risks are associated with viruses, transforming proteins, DNA and the characteristics of the producer cell line.

5.1 Viruses

The presence of endogenous viruses associated with a cell line poses a recognizable risk for product contamination. Retroviruses are of particular concern because of their tumorigenic potential. For many processes, a variety of chemical and physical treatments during product isolation may be sufficient to inactivate any contaminating viruses. However, in order to be certain, it is essential to validate the efficiency of the purification process by following the loss of viability of a range of known viruses added at various stages of isolation. Viral assays may be performed to detect the presence of

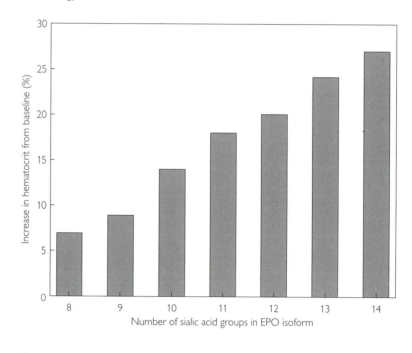

Figure 12.15

The biological activity of each isoform of EPO after a 30-day treatment.

contamination in the cell line, culture medium or serum used in the production process (Poiley, 1987). A wide margin of safety should be established in any inactivation process to ensure the elimination of all residual viral activity.

5.2   Transforming proteins

Proteins that are products of oncogenes can act as growth factors in promoting cell division. Such growth factors may be secreted by the cells used in the production of biologicals and the risk of such proteins causing tumorigenesis has been considered. However, these proteins are rapidly inactivated when administered *in vivo* and unlike other contaminating agents they have no potential for replication.

The growth-promoting effects of these factors are transient and reversible. The transforming agent would have to be synthesized continuously to maintain a transformed cell. Thus, even if co-purified with the required biological product, such contaminating proteins would be incapable of causing or maintaining the transformation of cells *in vivo*. Consequently no specific tests are considered necessary to ensure their elimination. The high purity of the final product is generally regarded as a sufficient safeguard against the risk of such contaminating proteins.

5.3   Residual cellular DNA

The DNA content of animal cell-derived therapeutic products causes the greatest concern because of the potential for carrying fragments of oncogenes. The oncogenes may have the potential for replication and could lead to tumorigenesis. These genes are expressed in cancer cells and ensure their continuous growth potential. In order to eliminate the risk of product contamination with oncogenes, the purification process should reduce the residual DNA content to a minimal and safe level.

Current methods of analysis allow the determination of residual DNA in an isolated cell culture product to a concentration of at least 1 pg/ml. A DNA content of <10 pg/dose of an injectable product is sufficiently low to assess the risk of tumorigenesis as negligible. This level of DNA is several orders of magnitude lower than the minimum required for cell transformation *in vitro*.

5.4   Safety of the cell line

Although continuous cell lines have good growth characteristics in large-scale culture, they were restricted from use in licensed production processes for many years because of the perceived risk of transmission of tumorigenic agents. These cell lines are known to have activated oncogenes and many harbor endogenous viruses. However, the extensive characterization of certain cell lines and the ability to reduce the detection limits of known contaminants such as DNA has enabled a relaxation of the blanket restriction against the use of these cells. Greater emphasis has now been placed on the ability to prove that the final products are not contaminated and are therefore risk-free.

In the case of production of recombinant proteins it is essential to use continuous cell lines. Protocols for genetic engineering require continuous cell culture for over 100 population doublings before a suitable high-producing cell line is obtained. Normal diploid cell lines would enter the senescence state well before such procedures were complete. Many recombinant products from continuous cell lines have been accepted for clinical use and approval is related to the maintenance of stringent procedures of culture and product purification.

6.   Tissue engineering

The ability to re-constitute human tissue from combinations of cell types grown in culture is an important prospect for future therapeutic treatment associated with organ failure (Stock and Vacanti, 2001). Up to now the most successful application of tissue engineering is in the re-constitution of skin following severe burns.

6.1   Artificial skin

The reconstitution of human tissue is important for skin grafting (Schulz *et al.*, 2000). Artificial skin can be formed from two layers derived from cultured human cells (Hardin-Young and Parenteau, 2002):

■   a dermal-equivalent formed from fibroblasts;
■   an epidermal-equivalent which is layered on the dermal surface.

To construct a dermal-equivalent, fibroblasts are dissociated from a tissue biopsy and mixed with predetermined proportions of collagen in culture medium. The mixture is poured into a mold, the shape of which determines the geometry of the constructed tissue. The fibroblasts cause the condensation of the collagen into fibrils to form a gel-like matrix which excludes most of the surrounding fluid. During a 6-day culture period the cells attach to the collagen forming a contracted matrix of tissue-like consistency.

An epidermal-equivalent developed from keratinocytes is then layered on the surface of the dermal-equivalent. The epidermal cells attach to the collagen substratum to form a continuous sheet in which cells can differentiate and form multilayers. After 10 days the epidermal cells may be exposed to air to allow the formation of an outer protective layer (stratum corneum) which consists of a layer of dead cells. The bi-layer of cells increases in thickness over time and results in a controlled deposition of matrix proteins.

This living bi-layered skin substitute is created to heal wounds and has been used successfully for grafting to burns patients. The process has been demonstrated to be safe and effective for therapeutic treatment. Clinical trials of one such product (Apligraf from Organogenesis Inc.) has been effective in the treatment of acute and chronic wounds without immunosuppressive therapy.

The keratinocytes and fibroblasts are derived from neonatal foreskin tissue and lack antigen presentation that would cause an adverse immune response. The skin substitute can be cryopreserved under liquid nitrogen and reconstituted quickly when required.

6.2   Artificial organs

Attempts to construct organs other than skin equivalents have met greater technical difficulties. Multiple cell types require more complex scaffolds and an extracellular matrix to support the functional relationship between cells. A further level of complexity is that multiple cell layers require a nutrient supply equivalent to blood capillaries *in vivo*.

However, the use of cultured cells to replace damaged cells *in vivo* offers some immediate and promising possibilities. This concept has been developed for pancreatic cells capable of secreting insulin to replace damaged islet cells in patients with diabetes (Lim and Sun, 1980). One problem is how to protect the transplanted cells from immunogenic rejection. A possible solution is to encapsulate the cells in a matrix such as alginate or agarose (see Chapter 10). This would protect the cells from immunological rejection but still allow the free flow of nutrients and small secreted cell products. Thus, hormone replacement therapy may be possible by development of such artificial organs.

7.   Cells as products

This section describes the various ways that cells can be useful in procedures for toxicity testing and for various clinical or therapeutic applications.

7.1   Drug screening and toxicity tests

The use of whole animal tests to establish the potential toxicity of compounds has been routine for many years. However, there are a number of disadvantages and objections to the continuation of these tests. The cost and variability of results is considerable. Also, there are growing moral objections to the use of animals for such purposes.

Mammalian cell cultures can offer the basis for alternative test systems that may overcome some of these disadvantages (Balls *et al.*, 1991). Cell culture tests are rapid, allow more efficient screening of novel compounds and sometimes can allow the identification of metabolic targets of inhibition. These test systems can be designed to evaluate various effects:

- reduced growth rate;
- breakdown of membrane permeability;
- tissue specificity of response;
- ability to metabolize toxic compounds;
- simulated wound healing;
- damage repair by use of artificially constructed tissue;
- genetic effects/mutagenicity, i.e. interaction with DNA.

7.2   Cell therapy

The ability to expand and differentiate hematopoietic stem cells *ex vivo* as described in Chapter 2 has many clinical applications (Nielsen, 1999). There is a high turnover of hematopoietic cells *in vivo* as a result of continuous growth and replacement. This makes the cells vulnerable to destruction by any cytotoxic drugs used in chemotherapy to eradicate residual tumor cells. Removal of bone marrow cells prior to chemotherapy allows isolation and expansion of the pluripotent stem cells to provide a source of mature hematopoietic cells following chemotherapy.

The *ex vivo* cell expansion can be manipulated by careful culture control of stem cells to allow the production of a cell population enriched with specific cells lines. This procedure can be useful for the production of specific T-lymphocytes or natural killer cells that may be required for cell-mediated immunotherapy. The hematopoietic stem cells can also be an appropriate target for somatic gene therapy as described in the next section.

It is often difficult to identify the stem cells from a mixed population, although one method that has been widely adopted is immunopurification with anti-CD34 antibodies. The cell population isolated with a cell surface CD34 antigen is enriched with hematopoietic stem cells. These can be expanded in a medium containing a controlled balance of cytokines. It has been found that various cell culture parameters including oxygen, pH, osmolarity and cytokine composition can influence the extent and direction of differentiation.

7.3   Gene therapy

The development of methods for transfecting exogenous genes into mammalian cells (see Chapter 6) has been extremely important for producing cells capable of expressing large quantities of therapeutic proteins in culture. However, the transfected cells themselves may also be used directly as a treatment for certain genetic diseases associated with inborn errors of metabolism.

The concept of gene therapy is that a missing or faulty gene is replaced by a normal, working gene. The process involves the transfection of a specific gene into cells of a patient with an identified and well-characterized genetic disease. The gene can be introduced into cells inside the patient (*in vivo*) or outside the patient (*ex vivo*). For the *ex vivo* process the cells that are removed are then re-introduced into the patient when they express the normal protein which alleviates the metabolic defect (*Figure 12.16*).

An example of the successful application of this is in the treatment of severe combined immunodeficiency (SCID) associated with a defective copy

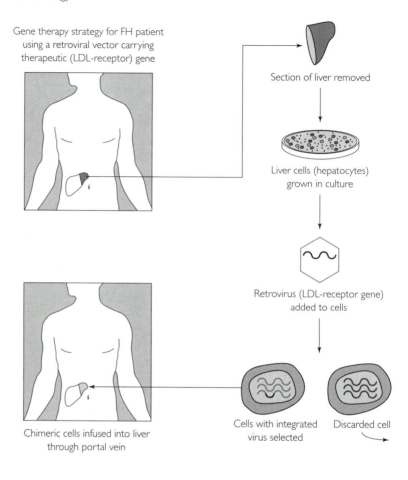

Gene therapy strategy for FH patient using a retroviral vector carrying therapeutic (LDL-receptor) gene

Section of liver removed

Liver cells (hepatocytes) grown in culture

Retrovirus (LDL-receptor gene) added to cells

Cells with integrated virus selected   Discarded cell

Chimeric cells infused into liver through portal vein

Figure 12.16

The principle of gene therapy ex vivo. *FH, familial hypercholesterolemia; LDL, low-density lipoprotein.*

of a gene on the X-chromosome required for the expression of the enzyme adenosine deaminase (ADA). Treatment by gene therapy involves the isolation of bone marrow stem cells from the patient followed by *in vitro* infection of the cells with a retrovirus constructed to carry the ADA gene. The transduced stem cells are then re-introduced into the bone marrow of the patient where they can proliferate and differentiate into immunocompetent cells. This treatment has been carried out on a small number of patients.

Treatment of this type may be applied to other diseases associated with bloodborne cells. For example, the therapeutic procedure is suitable for treatment of disorders associated with hemoglobin, such as sickle cell anemia or thalassemia. Sickle cell anemia arises from a single point mutation in the β-globin gene. The thalassemias represent a collection of globin abnormalities, arising from a reduction in α-chain synthesis (α-thalassemia) or in β-chain synthesis (β-thalassemia). The hematopoietic cells can be isolated from the bone marrow and transfected with normal globin genes using retroviral vectors. These cells when re-introduced into the bone marrow will provide a continuous source of normal hemoglobin (Noll *et al.*, 2002).

Other potential disease targets for gene therapy include Lesch-Nyhan syndrome, which is an X-linked recessive deficiency of the hypoxanthine-guanine phosphoribosyltransferase (HGPRT) enzyme and phenylketonuria, which is associated with deficient phenylalanine hydroxylase enzyme. There is some debate as to the most effective and safe vector to be used in gene therapy. There are two perceived dangers:

■   there may be a severe immune reaction to the applied viral vector;
■   the viral vector may integrate into the DNA of a cell in a way to cause the activation of a cellular proto-oncogene.

The four viral vectors that have been considered for gene therapy are:

■   retroviruses;
■   adenoviruses;
■   adeno-associated viruses;
■   herpes simplex virus.

These viruses vary in their characteristics and requirements (*Table 12.3*). The ideal viral vector shows efficient entry into cells followed by high gene expression for long periods. None of these vector types is ideal in all situations.

8. Conclusion

The number of novel recombinant proteins to have received regulatory approval as human therapeutic agents has risen sharply in the last few years (*Figure 12.17*). As a result of opportunities arising from the human genome project, an understanding of the role of specific genes has given rise to a large number of potential mammalian proteins to be used as therapeutic agents. At the present time more than 200 drugs derived from mammalian cell cultures are in clinical trials, and about 70 of those drugs are expected to come

Table 12.3. Advantages and disadvantages of different viral vectors

Vector	Advantages	Disadvantages
Retrovirus	– enters cells efficiently – viral genes absent – integrates stably into genome	– difficult to produce – limited insert size – random mutagenesis
Adenovirus	– enters cells efficiently – produces high expression – does not integrate into genome	– viral genes in vector – induces immune response
Adeno-associated virus	– integrates at specific sites – does not produce immune response	– small insert – difficult to produce
Herpes virus	– produced at high levels – targets nondividing nerve cells	– difficult to produce – viral genes required

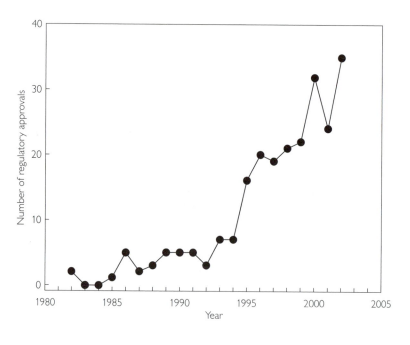

Figure 12.17

New biotechnology drug and vaccine approvals per year.

to market by 2006. A high proportion of these are humanized monoclonal antibodies and many are targeted as anticancer agents.

The need to produce this large number of glycoproteins under GMP (Good Manufacturing Practice) conditions will result in enormous pressure on the available manufacturing facilities. There is a well-recognized shortage of pharmaceutical and contract manufacturing facilities for the large-scale production of the recombinant protein products targeted as potential thera-peutic agents. The current worldwide cell culture capacity, estimated at 450 000 liters, is almost fully utilized. To meet this demand biopharmaceu-tical companies and contract manufacturers are now attempting to triple their production capacity. However, new bioprocessing plants take 3–5 years to design, build, and certify. This has already resulted in shortfalls in pro-duction. For example, it is reported that the lack of manufacturing capacity for the biopharmaceutical company, Immunex, resulted in a loss of revenue of more than $200 million for its arthritis drug in 2001 (Mallik *et al.*, 2002).

The cost efficiency of a production process becomes more important as products move out of the patented domain of specific companies. Competition amongst generic recombinant protein producers will force a concerted effort for low-cost production. An example of this is the commer-cial production of EPO. Amgen's production process for this therapeutic protein is an inefficient multiple-culture system based on roller bottles. The lack of process control leads to the recovery of only 20% of an appropriately glycosylated product. Patent protection presently enables Amgen to recover costs despite this inefficiency. However, as the patent period for EPO is coming to an end so generic manufacturers are designing cost-efficient bioprocesses that will allow profitability in a more competitive market.

There will be increased pressure to obtain skilled manpower that will allow the development of an increased capacity for production. The biopharmaceutical industry faces a looming shortage of the highly trained people needed to design, build, and operate manufacturing facilities. Experienced process-development scientists and engineers, validation engineers, quality assurance personnel, and plant managers are already in short supply. Universities are not producing anywhere near as many qualified manufacturing specialists as the industry needs. The number of graduate students enrolled in biology, cell biology, biochemistry, and chemical engineering programs has remained flat, whereas demand has increased with the addition of new capacity (Mallik *et al.*, 2002).

These developments will ensure the importance of animal cell technology in the future and it is hoped that the contents of this book will educate and inspire future practitioners of these bioprocesses.

References

Anson, D.S., Austen, D.E.G. and Brownlee, G.G. (1985) Expression of active human clotting factor IX from recombinant DNA clones in mammalian cells. *Nature* **315**: 683–685.

Balls, M., Garle, M. and Clothier, R.H. (eds) (1991) Future developments in in vitro methodology. In: *Animals and Alternatives in Toxicology – Present Status and Future Prospects*, pp. 313–339. Macmillan Press, London.

Brickelmaier, M., Hochman, P.S., Baciu, R., Chao, B., Cuervo, J.H. and Whitty, A. (1999) ELISA methods for the analysis of antibody responses induced in multiple sclerosis patients treated with recombinant interferon-beta. *J. Immunol. Methods* **227**: 121–135.

Clark, J.M. and Hirtenstein, M.D. (1981) High yield culture of human fibroblasts on microcarriers: a first step in production of fibroblast-derived interferon (human beta interferon). *J. Interferon Res.* **1**: 391–400.

Conradt, H.S., Egge, H., Peter-Katalinic, J., Reiser, W., Siklosi, T. and Schaper, K. (1987) Structure of the carbohydrate moiety of human interferon-beta secreted by a recombinant Chinese hamster ovary cell line. *J. Biol. Chem.* **262**: 14600–14605.

Egrie, J.C. and Browne, J.K. (2001) Development and characterization of novel erythropoiesis stimulating protein (NESP). *Br. J. Cancer* **84** (Suppl 1): 3–10.

Eridani, S. (1990) Erythropoietin. In: Spier R.E. and Griffiths, J.E. (eds) *Animal Cell Biotechnology*, Vol. 4, pp. 475–491. Academic Press, London.

Goto, M., Akai, K., Murakami, A. *et al.* (1988) Production of recombinant human erythropoietin in mammalian cells: host-cell dependency of the biological activity of the cloned glycoprotein. *Biotechnology* **6**: 67–71.

Hardin-Young, J. and Parenteau, N.L. (2002) Bilayered skin constructs. In: Atala and Lanza, R.P. (eds) *Methods of Tissue Engineering*, pp. 1177–1188. Academic Press, London.

Isaacs, A. and Lindenmann, J. (1957) Viral interference 1. The interferon. *Proc. R. Soc.* **147**: 258.

James, K. (1990) Therapeutic monoclonal antibodies – their production and application. In: Spier, R.E. and Griffiths, J.B. (eds) *Animal Cell Biotechnology*, Vol. 4, pp. 205–255. Academic Press, London.

Kagawa, Y., Takasaki, S., Utsumi, J., Hosoi, K., Shimizu, H., Kochibe, N. and Kobata, A. (1988) Comparative study of the asparagine-linked sugar chains of natural human interferon-beta 1 and recombinant human interferon-beta 1 produced by three different mammalian cells. *J. Biol. Chem.* **263**: 17508–17515.

Lawn, R.M. and Vehar, G.A. (1986) The molecular genetics of haemophilia. *Sci. Am.* **254**: 40–46.

Lazar, A. (1983) Interferon production by human lymphoblastoid cells. *Adv. Biotechnol. Proc.* **2**: 179–208.

Lim, F. and Sun, A.M. (1980) Microencapsulated islets as bioartificial endocrine pancreas. *Science* **120**: 908–910.

Lubiniecki, A.S. (1987) Continuous cell substrate considerations. In: Lubiniecki A.S. (ed.) *Large-Scale Mammalian Cell Culture Technology*, pp. 495–513. Marcel Dekker, New York.

Lubiniecki, A.S. and Lupker, J.H. (1994) Purified protein products of rDNA technology expressed in animal cell culture. *Biologicals* **22**: 161–169.

Lubiniecki, A.S., Arathoon, R., Polastri, G., Thomas, J., Wiebe, M., Garnick, R., Jones, A., van Reis, R. and Builder, S.E. (1989) Selected strategies for manufacture and control of recombinant tissue plasminogen activator prepared from cell cultures. In: Spiers, R.E., Griffiths, J.B., Stephenne, J. *et al.* (eds) *Advances in Animal Cell Biology and Technology for Bioprocesses*, pp. 442–451. Butterworth, Oxford.

Mahy, B.W.J. (1985) *Virology: A Practical Approach*. IRL Press, Oxford.

Mallik, A., Pinkus, G.S. and Sheffer, S. (2002) Biopharma's capacity crunch. *The McKinsey Quarterly* Special Edition on 'Risk and Resilience' 9–11.

Nielsen, L.K. (1999) Bioreactors for hematopoietic cell culture. *Annu. Rev. Biomed. Eng.* **1**: 129–152.

Noll, T., Jelinek, N., Schmid, S., Biselli, M. and Wandrey, C. (2002) Cultivation of hematopoietic stem and progenitor cells: biochemical engineering aspects. *Adv. Biochem. Eng. Biotechnol.* **74**: 111–128.

Petricciani, J.C. (1987) Should continuous cell lines be used as substrates for biological products? *Dev. Biol. Stand.* **66**: 3–12.

Poiley, J.A. (1987) Methods for the detection of adventitious viruses in cell cultures used in the production of biotechnology products. In: Lubiniecki, A.S. (ed.) *Large-Scale Mammalian Cell Culture Technology*, pp. 483–494. Marcel Dekker, New York.

Qin, X.Q., Tao, N., Dergay, A., Moy, P., Fawell, S., Davis, A., Wilson, J.M. and Barsoum, J. (1998) Interferon-beta gene therapy inhibits tumor formation and causes regression of established tumors in immune-deficient mice. *Proc. Natl Acad. Sci. USA* **95**: 14411–14416.

Runkel, L., Meier, W., Pepinsky, R.B. *et al.* (1998) Structural and functional differences between glycosylated and non-glycosylated forms of human interferon-beta (IFN-beta). *Pharm. Res.* **15**: 641–649.

Scahill, S.J., Devos, R., van der Heyden, J. and Fiers, W. (1983) Expression and characterization of the product of a human immune interferon cDNA gene in Chinese hamster ovary cells. *Proc. Natl. Acad. Sci. USA* **80**: 4654–4658.

Schulz, J.T., Tompkins, R.G. and Burke, J.F. (2000) Artificial skin. *Ann. Rev. Med.* **51**: 231–244.

Stock, U.A. and Vacanti, J.P. (2001) Tissue engineering: current state and prospects. *Ann. Rev. Med.* **52**: 443–451.

von Mehren, M., Adams, G.P. and Weiner, L.M. (2003) Monoclonal antibody therapy for cancer. *Ann. Rev. Med.* **54**: 343–369.

Wood, W.I., Capon, D.J., Simonsen, C.C. *et al.* (1984) Expression of active human factor VIII from recombinant DNA clones. *Nature* **312**: 330–337.

Further reading

Aiuti, A., Slavin, S. and Aker, M. (2002) Correction of ADA-SCID by stem cell gene therapy combined with nonmyeloablative conditioning. *Science* **296**: 2410–2413.

Bianco, P. and Robey, P.G. (2001) Stem cells in tissue engineering. *Nature* **414**: 118–121.

Buckley, R.H. (2002) Gene theapy for SCID – a complication after remarkable progress. *Lancet* (North American edition) **360**: 1185–1186.

Friedman, R.M. (1981) *Interferons – a primer*. Academic Press, New York.

Handgretinger, R., Cavazzana-Calvo, M. and Hacein-Bey-Abina, S. (2002) Gene therapy for severe combined immunodeficiency disease. *New Engl. J. Med.* **347**: 613–614.

Kaji, E.H. and Leiden, J.M. (2001) Gene and stem cell therapies. *JAMA* **285**: 545–550.

Kluft, C. *et al.* (1983) Large-scale production of extrinsic (tissue-type) plasminogen activators from human melanoma cells. *Adv. Biotechnol. Processes* **2**: 97–110.

Larrick, J.W. and Burck, K.L. (1991) *Gene Therapy: Application of Molecular Biology.* Elsevier, New York.

Lerner, R.A. (1983) Synthetic vaccines. *Sci. Am.* **248**: 48–56.

Mizrahi, A., Lazar, A. and Reuveny, S. (1990) Interferons derived from human cells. In: Spier, R.E. and Griffiths, J.B. (eds) *Animal Cell Biotechnology*, Vol. 4, pp. 413–444. Academic Press, London.

Noguchi, P. (2003) Risks and benefits of gene therapy. *New Engl. J. Med.* **348**: 193–194.

Panem, S. (1984) *The Interferon Crusade.* Brookings Institute, Washington.

Peake, I.R. (1985) Molecular biology of blood coagulation disorders. *Bioessays* **2**: 110–113.

Plotkin, S.A. and Mortimer, M.D. Jr. (1988) *Vaccines.* W.B. Saunders, Philadelphia.

Seppa, N. (2001) Gene therapy for sickle-cell disease? *Science News* **160**: 372.

Stones, P.B. (1981) *Viral Vaccines. Essays in Applied Microbiology.* J.Wiley, London.

Wilmut, I. (1998) Cloning for medicine. *Sci. Am.* **279**: 58–63.

Woodrow, G.C. and Levine, M.M. (1990) *New Generation Vaccines.* Marcel Dekker, New York.

Zandstra, P.W. and Nagy, A. (2001) Stem cell bioengineering. *Annu. Rev. Biomed. Eng.* **3**: 275–305.

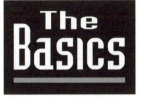

Glossary

Adaptation	Metabolic changes that occur when cells are introduced into a new culture medium. This may involve induction or repression of specific enzymes.
Anchorage-dependent cells	Cells that require a solid surface for attachment and growth.
Aneuploid	A cell having a chromosome number different from a multiple of the haploid number.
Antibody	A glycoprotein released by a B-lymphocyte in response to a foreign compound (antigen). The antibody can bind to the antigen.
Antigen	A compound that induces the formation of a specific antibody.
Apoptosis	Cell death caused by the activation of intracellular degradative enzymes. This is akin to a 'suicide mechanism' for cells.
Aseptic	Free of microorganisms.
Attenuation	A term used in the context of vaccines – to make an immunogenic but nonpathogenic virus.
Autoradiography	Detection of radioactive material by exposure to X-ray film.
Biological	A commercially useful product from cells. It may be a single compound or a complex mixture.
Bioreactor	A vessel (or fermenter) capable of supporting a cell culture typically to a large scale.
Capsid	The protein coat that encloses the nucleic acid of a virus.
Carcinogenesis	The generation of cancer cells.
Cell culture	The growth of cells as independent units. The cells are not organized as in tissues.
Cell cycle	The phases through which cells proceed during growth (G1 – S – G2 – M).
Cell fusion (or hybridization)	The process of two cells fusing (or hybridizing) into one. This can be induced by viruses or chemicals known as fusogens or by an electric field of high intensity. The resulting fused cell is called a heterokaryon and might be quite unstable genetically.
Cell hybridization (or fusion)	The fusion of two or more dissimilar cells. See cell fusion.

Cell line	Cells that originate by subculture of a primary culture. The term may be prefixed by 'finite' or 'continuous' to indicate the potential for further subculture.
Cell strain	Cells derived from a cell line or primary culture by selection of a specific property or marker which is maintained through subsequent subcultures. Usually, selection of the cell strain is carried out by cloning.
Chemostat	Continuous culture in which the cells flow out of the fermenter with the effluent. The growth rate is governed by the rate of supply of a limiting nutrient in the supplied medium.
Clone	A population of genetically identical cells derived from an individual cell.
Collagen	A proteolytic enzyme specific for the breakdown of collagen.
Complementary DNA (cDNA)	DNA formed by reverse transcription of mRNA.
Confluent	The point of maximum cell density arising through exhaustion of culture medium or the complete cover of the available growth surface.
Constant region	The region of an immunoglobulin in which the amino acid sequence does not show changes within a given antibody isotype.
Continuous cell line	A cell population having an infinite capacity for growth. Often referred to as 'immortal' and previously referred to as 'established'.
Coulter counter	An electronic particle counter that can be used to determine the concentration of cells in a culture sample.
Cryopreservation	The maintenance of cells in a frozen state – usually in liquid nitrogen.
Cryopreservative	Compounds which prevent cell damage during the freezing and thawing associated with cryopreservation, e.g. glycerol or dimethylsulfoxide (DMSO).
Differentiated	Cells which have become specialized for a particular function.
Diploid	The state of a cell in which chromosomes (except sex chromosomes) are paired and are structurally identical with those of the species from which they were derived. Each species has a characteristic number of chromosomes in the diploid state (e.g. human = 46).
Doubling time	The time (h) taken for a cell population to double in number.
Downstream processing	The process of extraction and purification of a product from cell culture.
Electrofusion	The application of electrical impulses to cause cell fusion.

Electroporation	The exposure of cells to an electrical impulse to allow the uptake of DNA.
Enzyme-linked immunosorbent assay (ELISA)	An assay used to measure the concentration of an antigen or antibody.
Epithelial cell	A cell type derived from epithelia, which is a layer covering an internal or external surface.
Explant	A tissue taken from an animal and transferred to culture medium.
Fibroblast	A cell type found in connective tissue in association with collagen.
Flow cytometer	An instrument capable of distinguishing cells labeled with a fluorescent marker – used to determine the distribution of cells through the cell cycle.
Fluidized-bed (bio)reactor	A fermenter in which immobilized cells are agitated by a fluid flow of culture medium.
Fusogen	A substance that will cause the fusion of two cells.
Generation time (or doubling time)	The time interval between consecutive cell divisions. Typical values for an animal cell population are 20–24 h.
Genome	The complete set of genes of an organism.
Genotype	The total genetic characteristics of a cell.
Glycosylation	The metabolic pathway found in eukaryotic cells that allows the addition of a carbohydrate group on to a protein.
Growth curve	A graphical plot of cell concentration (often a log scale) against time (linear scale) during growth of a cell culture. The curve can be divided into lag, log and stationary phase.
Growth cycle	The period during cell culture from subculture to the end of exponential growth.
Haploid	Describes the state of germ cells after meiosis when each chromosome is represented once.
Hayflick limit	The finite number of generations that a normal cell can grow.
HeLa	A human cell line derived from a cervical cancer of a patient in 1953 named Henrietta Lach.
Hemocytometer	A glass microscope slide marked with a grid that can be used to determine the number of cells in a set volume.
HEPA	High-efficiency particulate air filters used in laminar flow cabinets to filter the air supply.
Hepatocyte	A liver cell.
Heterokaryon	A cell possessing two or more genetically different nuclei in a common cytoplasm. This state arises following cell fusion.
Heteroploid	A term used to describe a cell culture that contains cells having chromosome numbers other than the diploid number.

Hollow-fiber (bio)reactor	A culture system consisting of a bundle of semi-permeable hollow fibers.
Human anti-murine antibody (HAMA)	This is produced as a human immune response to a mouse antibody.
Hybrid cell	A mononucleate cell resulting from the fusion of two cells.
Hybridoma	A stable hybrid cell that secretes a monoclonal antibody. The hybridoma is created from the fusion of an antibody-secreting B-lymphocyte and a transformed myeloma. The term was first used in the 1970s following the breakthrough work of Kohler and Milstein.
Immortalization	The transformation of a cell with a finite life-span to one possessing an infinite lifespan.
Immunoglobulin	Proteins found in the blood. They show antibody activity.
Interleukin	One of a group of compounds acting between leukocytes and capable of a variety of stimulatory activity.
Isotonic	A culture medium, the osmotic pressure of which is the same as intracellular fluid.
Karyotype	The chromosomal complement of a cell.
Keratinocyte	Cell of the epithelium that synthesizes keratin.
Lag phase	The period after subculture of cells but before growth is fully established. This period is associated with the adaptation of cells to new conditions.
Laminar flow cabinet	A sterile work station consisting of a filtered air flow.
Leukocyte (or leucocyte)	A white blood cell.
Lipofection	Incorporation of DNA into a cell using liposomes.
Liposome	A complex of charged lipids and DNA that can be readily incorporated into cells.
Log phase	The period during culture of active cell growth. This is also known as the exponential phase.
Lymphoblast	A lymphocyte which has been stimulated to divide by an antigen.
Lymphoblastoid	A transformed lymphoblast capable of infinite growth capacity.
Lymphocyte	A nongranular type of white blood cell. There are two forms: the T-lymphocyte and the B-lymphocyte.
Lymphokine	One of a group of compounds released by lymphocytes and causing a variety of stimulatory activity.
Malignant	Describes a tumor which has become invasive (metastatic), i.e. capable of colonizing other tissues.

Microcarrier	A microscopic particle capable of supporting cell attachment and growth of anchorage-dependent cells.
Mitogen	A compound capable of inducing mitosis.
Mitosis	Cell division by which two new cells have the same genetic content as the parent.
Monoclonal	From a population of cells which is derived from one cell (a clone).
Monoclonal antibody	An antibody that is specific to a single antigen. A monoclonal antibody is synthesized from a homogeneous population of hybridoma cells.
Mutagen	An agent (mutagenic compound) that causes a mutation.
Mutant	A phenotypic variant cell resulting from an altered gene.
Myeloma	A tumor cell derived from a B-lymphocyte and capable of continuous growth (also known as a plasmacytoma).
Mycoplasma	Gram-negative bacteria that can grow within the animal cell cytoplasm.
Necrosis	Cell death associated with a sudden severe insult or stress. This usually occurs by breakdown of the plasma membrane leading to cell swelling and rupture.
Nonanchorage-dependent cells	Cells that can be grown in suspension without the need of a solid support.
Oncogene	A gene that is active in transformed cells.
Organ culture	The maintenance or growth of the whole or part of an organ *in vitro*. The differentiation of the cells and the tissue architecture is preserved.
Osmolarity	A measure of osmotic pressure of culture media expressed as the molarity of dissociated particles – typically around 300 mOsm/liter.
Osmometer	An instrument to measure the osmolarity of a liquid, usually by the depression of the freezing point compared to a standard (distilled water).
Packed-bed (bio)reactor	A fermenter consisting of a static bed of beads containing immobilized cells.
Passage (or subculture)	The transfer of cells from one culture vessel to another. Usually this is accompanied by a dilution of the cell concentration.
Passage number	The number of subcultures (or passages) performed after the original isolation of the cells from a primary source.
Perfusion	Continuous culture in which cells are retained in the fermenter.
PID control	Proportional, integral and derivative control used to minimize changes from a set point in a culture. Commonly applied to maintain a constant pH or dissolved oxygen at a preset value.

Plating efficiency	The ability of cell population to form colonies and is expressed as the percentage of cells inoculated into a culture vessel that give rise to discrete colonies.
Pluripotent	The capacity of an embryonic cell to differentiate to any cell type.
Pluronic	A polymer commonly added to culture media to reduce damage to cells by gas sparging.
Polyethylene glycol	This is a commonly used fusogen for the fusion of two cells.
Population density	The number of cells per unit area of growth surface (in the case of anchorage-dependent cells) or per unit volume of culture.
Primary culture	A culture of cells taken directly from the tissue of an animal.
Quadroma	A cell formed by the fusion of two hybridomas. The immunoglobulin product of a quadroma will contain a mixture of heavy and light chain structures derived from each parental line.
Radioimmunoassay (RIA)	An assay to measure the concentration of an antigen or antibody by use of a radioactive label.
Recombinant product	A protein produced from a foreign DNA sequence introduced into a cell.
Retrovirus	RNA virus that replicates via conversion into a DNA duplex.
Roller bottle	A cylindrical vessel capable of supporting the growth of cells on its inner surface.
Serum-free medium	A culture medium in which serum has been replaced by a mixture of chemically defined components.
Split ratio	The number of new cultures established from a parent culture during subculture, e.g. if one culture flask is used to establish four new cultures, the split ratio is 4.
Stationary phase	The period in culture after the log phase of growth when cell division ceases.
Stirred tank (bio)reactor	A simple fermenter consisting of a cylindrical vessel with a stirrer.
Subculture	see Passage.
Substratum	The growth surface available for the attachment and growth of anchorage-dependent cells.
Suspension culture	A culture consisting of cells suspended in the liquid culture medium.
T-flask	A flat-based (tissue culture) flask capable of supporting the growth of cells.
T-lymphocyte	Cells derived from the thymus and capable of cell-mediated immunity.
Telomere	Repeated nucleotide sequence at the end of a chromosome. The sequence shortens during mitosis of normal cells.

Teratoma	A mass of several cell types formed from an embryonic stem cell.
Tissue culture	The maintenance or growth of tissues *in vitro* with the preservation of the differentiated cells and the integrity of the intercellular arrangement and architecture.
Transfection	The transfer of genetic material into animal cells. The term 'transformation' is used for such a process in bacteria.
Transformation	The conversion of a normal eukaryotic cell to one with the ability for continuous growth in culture. The term is also applied to the incorporation of genetic material into prokaryotic cells.
Trypsin	A proteolytic enzyme required to remove anchorage-dependent cells from their attached substratum.
Tumorigenic	Giving rise to a tumor.
Ultrafiltration	Filtration under pressure used to concentrate culture medium as a preliminary to product extraction.
Variable region	The region of an immunoglobulin in which the amino acid sequence changes so that the molecule can bind to a specific antigen.
Viability	A measure of the proportion of live cells in a population.
Zymogram	An electrophoretic banding pattern of an isozyme. This is used to determine the species of origin of a cell line.

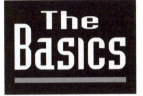

Index